MICHAEL HONE

MALE
SELF-PLEASURING

FROM DIOGENES TO FLESHLIGHTS

Cover painting detail of *John the Baptist* by da Vinci

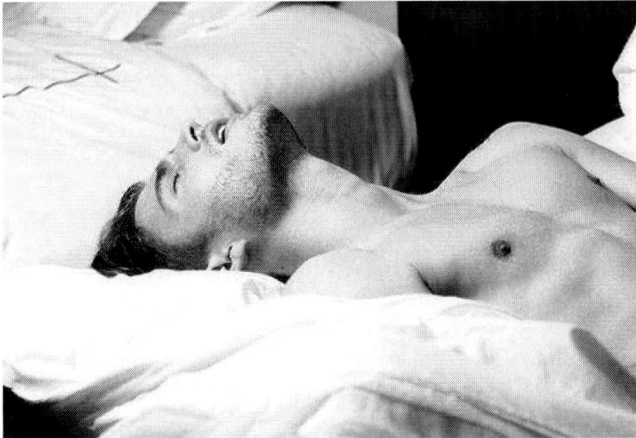

Masturbation is Healthy Pleasure

© 2018

''The talk in the dormitories and studies was of the grossest character, with repulsive scenes of onanism, mutual masturbation and obscene orgies of naked boys in bed together. There was no refinement, just animal lust.''
John Addington Symonds

The first order that William Makepeace Thackeray received on his first day at school from a schoolmate was ''Come & frig me,'' he wrote later.

''An orgasm a day keeps the doctor away,'' stated a leaflet issued to students by the Sheffield National Health Service, adding that it should be supplemented by five portions of fruit and one veg per day, and 30 minutes of exercise three times a week.

Diogenes, the first man ever to claim to be a citizen of the world, said: ''Of the three appetites, food, drink and sex, sex is the easiest to fulfill as one need only rub oneself to obtain instant satisfaction.''

''Pleasure is in your own hands,'' was the slogan for the 2009 campaign of the Spanish socialist Extremadura government, which paid out $16,000 in brochures and workshops dedicated to ''sexual self-exploration and the discovery of self-pleasuring.''

''When my worries oppress my body, with my left hand I release my pent-up fluids.''
Ancient Pompeii graffiti

You're a liar if you say you don't masturbate, a fool if you say you do.
A modern-age aphorism

''You make use of your left-hand whore ... your only lover.''
Martial, Roman poet, 38 A.D.-104 A.D.

''The only thing about masturbation to be ashamed of, is doing it badly.''
Sigmund Freud

''It is a need, and when one is not driven by that need, it is always a sweet thing.''
Diderot, French Enlightenment philosopher

''One is never masturbated better than by oneself.''
Gérard de Nerval, French poet and writer.

''Don't knock masturbation. It's sex with someone you love.''
Woody Allen

''Masturbation: In the nineteenth century it was a disease; in the twentieth, it's a cure.''

Thomas Szasz, psychiatrist and psychoanalyst

''Masturbation is the thinking man's television.''
Christopher Hampton, playwright and film director

''To the lonely it is company; to the forsaken it is a friend; to the aged and to the impotent it is a benefactor. They that are penniless are yet rich, in that they still have this majestic diversion. There are times when I prefer it to sodomy.''
Julius Caesar

''I cannot describe what I owe to this gentle art.'
Robinson Crusoe

''None knows it but to love it; none name it but to praise.''
Mark Twain

''What's good about masturbation is that you don't have to get dressed for it.''
Truman Capote

''Love has often been ignored in histories of sexuality in part because it is the most elusive of the four-letter words.''
George Haggerty, writer

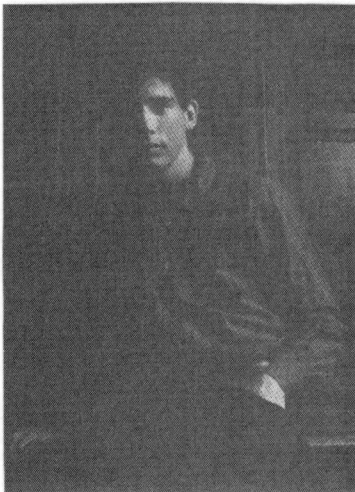

Photo of me taken in Paris, my life there related in my autobiography *Michael Hone: His World, His Loves.* My other books include: *Cellini* [a fully-revised 2018 edition], *Caravaggio* [a fully-revised 2018 edition], *Cesare Borgia, Renaissance Murders, TROY, Greek Homosexuality, ARGO, Alcibiades the Schoolboy, RENT BOYS, Buckingham, Homoerotic Art (in full color), Sailors and Homosexuality, The Essence of Being Gay, John (Jack) Nicholson, THE SACRED BAND, German Homosexuality, Gay*

Genius, SPARTA, Charles XII of Sweden, Mediterranean Homosexual Pleasure, CAPRI, Boarding School Homosexuality, American Homosexual Giants, HUSTLERS and *Christ has his John, I have my George: The History of British Homosexuality.* I live in the South of France.

<u>DEDICATION</u>

This book, on male pleasuring, is dedicated to a woman, Dr. Jocelyn Elders, fired by President Bill Clinton when she suggested that masturbation be taught in schools as a way of preventing young people from engaging in riskier forms of sex.

CHAPTER ONE

INTRODUCTION

The Masturbation Panic began precisely in 1760 and hit me personally full-force 200 years later, as found in this extract from my autobiography, *Michael Hone: His World, His Loves*: ''In the meantime there were physical and religious jolts, both dealing with the same subject. Rummaging around the grocery attic I came upon a 1910 medical journal. I looked up my favorite topic. There I read that my pastime was going to make me madder than a hatter. I went home in a daze. Now I knew the cause of my ill temper, my fits of despair, my parental disobedience. Everything fell neatly into place. I was evil because I was going insane. I was going insane because my brain was rotting. My brain was rotting because I gave myself pleasure. My hobby had been too good to be true. At home I confessed to my mother that I now knew why I was not the best little boy in the world--without going into details, of course, what boy could?--and promised to shape up.

''The solution--oh so simple--consisted of keeping my hands out of the vicinity of the troubling area. Three nights after promising Mother and God I would never do it again, I had only to rub--of so minutely, *à peine*, just the tiniest little bit--the extended pouch of his jockeys five harmless times again the bed sheets to bring on a heavenly bliss with full angelic and choral accompaniment. The resulting mess would not have pleased my mother who found me the cleanest of lads, but if this was madness, I was ready for the asylum. The discovery of this innocent stroking of cotton against cotton as-if-so-help-me-God-I-didn't-know-what-was-going-on was, as the French say, *le pied*, the foot, their expression for ecstasy.

''If incipient insanity was bad, offending God was worse still. As though one misfortune can't face life without another, the next Sunday a church speaker lowered the boom.

''A visiting bishop came into our all-male Mormon quorum to give us a little talk on sex, an unnerving proposition because the boys could not see what good a bishop could possibly have to say on the subject. The bishop, in his early twenties, was stooped and sparrow chested, bad form for a people whose creed was the Body is the Temple of the Spirit. If that was his temple, a gnat resided within. His face was chinless and sunfish narrow, and in his eyes burned the fire of martyrs. The way to damnation, he told us right off, passed through wicked hands. At the university, he went on, he had had a roommate who openly aroused himself on the adjoining bed. But the bishop had been there with a handy yardstick to whack the boy when the Devil got into those pouncing fingers. Bending over us like a bloodless Ichabod Crane, he spewed visions of bodies rotting in hell and brains open cesspools to death maggots. The boys shrank back as much from the ejected spit and clots of foam at the corners of his razor-thin liver-colored lips as from fear of the contagion of his own personal madness. Those boys, so bright and beautiful, wormed their backs into the plywood seats, a scorching heat burning into necks and ears, their throats so dry they had to cough to swallow. We who survived thanks to that sin, we who could stay the strain of continence because of it, who could overcome the pressures of exams, of growing up, of *being* thanks to it, we who would one day have families of our own, build our country, *die* for her, we were being warped by this shell of a human being whose inanities we swallowed. Terror was indeed catching, and we fell victim to it.

''Shackled spiritually and physically, I could only turn to God for help. I prayed day in and day out. I prayed until the tears streamed down my cheeks. But all He sent was cotton shorts against cotton sheets.

''That was the fissure that was to destroy my faith, the minuscule crevice through which the reservoir was to eventually burst.''

Not all the older boys and men who were guiding me through adolescence were Ichabod-Crane clones. Some were handsome athletes, serious in their advice as only Mormon-bred boys are capable of being, all of whom were obviously doing it on the sly, but none with the balls to admit it.

Lest the reader think that only redneck Utahns were afflicted, on the ship that brought me here to my adopted home, France, I had the great luck of meeting a Yale student who had promised his [Jewish] God that he would never jerk-off again, were he accepted through Yale's Pearly Gates [and what Heaven could possibly be as beautiful as the Yale campus?]. He was accepted by Yale, and kept the promise for an heroic three days, after which he counted, I imagine, on his God's forgiveness and understanding of the nature of boys.

Such were the consequences of the Masturbation Panic [to be thoroughly discussed], something certainly incomprehensible to the Internet boy of today.

CHAPTER TWO

MASTURBATION DURING ANTIQUITY

Egypt

Atum

It's surprising that so little of a self-pleasuring nature has come down to us from pharaonic times because the Egyptians recorded immense amounts of knowledge in the hieroglyphs they left behind.

We have the painting of Niânkhkhnoum and Khnoumhotep touching noses, the Egyptian kiss, taken as evident omnisexuality by some, an idea totally scoffed at by others.

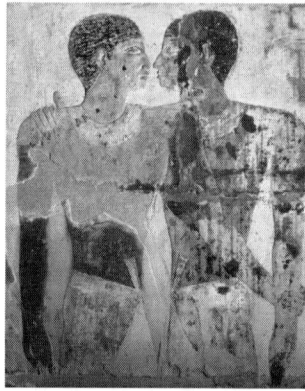

Niânkhkhnoum and Khnoumhotep, tenderly touching,
lovingly embracing.

In the Middle Kingdom King Pepi II regularly visited one of his soldiers, ''doing what he desires'', a text referring to an obvious homosexual liaison for some, a ridiculous assumption, state others. [The disagreements, perhaps in part, depend on which archeologists are heterosexual and which are homosexual.]

A documented papyrus concerning Seth and Horace is amusing and curious. Seth [the god of storms, chaos, desert and war] is jealous of Horus [god of the sky, war and hunting] because Horus is young and clearly favored by the others gods who appreciate his beauty. Seth decides to humiliate the boy by getting him drunk and ejaculating within him during a subsequent rape. Only, Horus has an inkling about what is going to take place and only pretends to drink. He does allow Seth to come in him, however, but then amasses the sperm that he puts on Seth's lettuce [lettuce considered an aphrodisiac by the Egyptians], that Seth eats the next day. Seth goes to Thot [judge and god of knowledge] to tell him that Horus allows himself to be taken. Thot then searches both men for semen. Seth's semen should normally come from the ass of Horus where Seth deposited it, but instead it comes out of Seth's own mouth. Horus is found innocent and Thot ponders how Seth's semen got inside himself.

Some archeologists maintain that this is proof of Seth's homosexuality [his taking Horus], while others say he performed the act only to humiliate Horus, especially as Seth had already tried to trick his sister into having intercourse, proof he was heterosexual.

Masturbation had immense importance for the Egyptians. The universe itself was created from the semen ejaculated by the Egyptian god Atum, the Nile itself the gift of his semen, its rise and fall directly tied to the frequency of Atum's ejaculates into the river. Each year, during the feast of Nim, pharaoh was ceremonially required to masturbate into the Nile, in recognition of Atum's creation of the universe, and to ensure and to nourish the river itself. He and his followers all stripped naked, and all approached close enough to the waters to ensure their fecundity, thanks to the ejaculations.

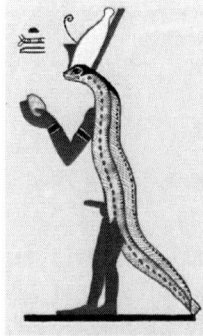

Atum, often represented as a serpent, a phallic symbol.
His first ejaculation was an attempt to lighten his loneliness and solitude, often the aim of masturbation today.

Through masturbation Atum gave birth to his children, who in turn gave birth to Osiris, Seth and Isis, which brings us back to the first paragraph of this chapter [more about Egyptian masturbation later].

Mesopotamia

Enki

Enki was the Lord of Earth, depicted with the Tigris and Euphrates springing from his shoulders, leaping with fish, whereas both rivers originated in his loins, which he gave birth to through masturbation. ''Enki lifted his eyes across the Euphrates and stood up full of lust like a rampant bull, lifted his penis, ejaculated and filled it with sweet flowing water, from which grew wine and barley to nourish the people. He lifted up his penis and filled the Tigris with more sweet water,'' from texts drawn from Sumerian literature.

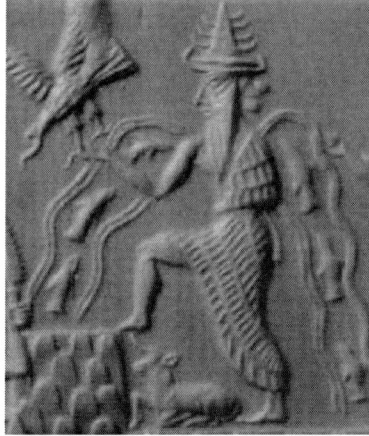

Enki.
Sumerians believed that masturbation enhanced sexual potency. Men often used *puru*-oil, a special oil probably mixed with pulverized iron ore intended to enhance friction.

Greece

Eros

The god who invented self-pleasuring was Eros, here in conversation with Helios, the Sun, and his sister Eos, the Dawn, she who rises red in the morning, blushing from the sight of young lovers in the throes of love, after a night of restoring sleep, an extract from my book *TROY*:

A handsome redheaded lad carrying a quiver on his back and a gold bow in his hand flew slowly towards them. Eros was of an age as yet untroubled by the havoc his arrows wrought, but he was amenable, as the poet said, to girls who would persuade him to play night games with them, laughing knowingly when he did as they asked.

"You look dog tired, adorable Eros," said Eos.

"I had a full night's work," smirked the god of Passion. "The weekends are really becoming insupportable. Orgies and onanism, secret assignations and happenstance encounters, bacchanals and banquets; not to speak of ordinary necking and necrophilia, seduction and sadism."

"I admire your handiwork, lovable Eros," said Helios. "And you're always so successful!"

"What god wouldn't be a success packing this quiver of love darts around? Is there a boy who does not awaken to my sting before his voice becomes that of a man? To my sting what maiden does not succumb to the lovesick eyes of her young pursuer? I am the eternal beginning, the everlasting renaissance, the glorious spring."

"Next you'll tell us that you're the most important of the gods," observed Eos.

"As the firstborn I have all the rights," scorned Eros, blood rushing to his ruddy cheeks. "In a family is not the first-born the most anticipated of children? Is he not the most ardent of a maiden's yearning and the great proof of her mate's virility? And when the first-born grows to manhood, is it not he, by law, who is responsible for his brothers and sisters and yea, must he not answer for the conduct of his mother and support her and her children and the household and servants and slaves when his father goes to war? Or if his father falls in battle, must he not take in charge his mother's and brothers' suitors and his sisters' dowries? Should he then not be the most respected and cuddled, the most honored and revered? Yes, say I."

"And I too, beautiful Eros," said Helios.

"As do I," seconded Eos. "We respect our little Eros, my brother and I. But we are in the minority. The other gods adore but do not adorn you. They think you--I hope you will not find this offensive and thereby wish to take revenge upon me--irresponsible, if not to say perverse."

"Oh! The ungrateful lot!" smoldered Eros.

"Perhaps, dearest Eros. No! Surely, I mean," said Helios,

redressing his awkwardness. "They surely are as you have said, ungrateful. And worse. Much worse. But wasn't it you and those love-tipped arrows of yours that brought forth from the union of Mother Earth and Tartarus the hideous god Typhon? Did you not push Thyestes to ravish Pelopia, his own daughter? Did not Apollo, mad with lust, take as lover Adonis--the first god to be united in ungodly lust with not only a mere mortal, but a boy?"

"As if you, Helios, did not crave for the sweet company of..."

"No, no, don't interrupt me, you wicked child!" Helios would have blushed were his coloring not already a brilliant gold. "What god is not driven to perversion by your silly whims and your ... your..." he sputtered, losing the thread of his thoughts. He ran his amber fingers through the bronze curls of his beard. "Where was I..."

"Adonis?" suggest Eos.

"Ah, yes. Thanks Sister. Adonis. And these are just some of the innumerable stories about your improprieties. Pushed by Passion, men have killed, shacked up with beasts, committed incest and have been driven to suicide. No horror is above your imagination, no abomination is beyond your capability, no sanctity is safe from your need to defile. In short, you're a scoundrel, darling Eros, a knave and a rascal, dearest, beautiful Eros."

"You wish me to be offended brother sun, but I'm thick-skinned and even if I did harbor some slight resentment against you, I would need but wait until you beg me for one of my favors without which you would spend your nights alone and loveless. I know that the gods--like the mortals--are ungrateful and never satisfied. All of you blame your woes on Eros, the first of the gods, for without me there would have been no inclination to produce others."

"How were you born, marvelous Eros?" inquired Eos. "It's been so long since I left school that I've totally forgotten the History of the Beginning of Time."

"My parents," began Eros, eager to take the stage, "were Mother Desire and Father Deviation, two old gods dethroned by the new ones. All I remember is awaking in the middle of a pile of egg shells where the ocean laps against the shore." In his mind's eye he saw the long crescent beach with its tepid sands and lucent waters. His birth had been a moment of such divine ecstasy that he carried its sweet imprint throughout the whole of his eventful, carefree life.

"And at birth you found yourself completely on your own?" asked Helios.

"Yes, and as a god I was full-grown when only nine days old. I was very curious and since I was alone, I had only myself to play with. One day, therefore, as I was taking in the warmth of a brilliant afternoon and pursuing solitary amusement in the hollow of some rocks a few feet above the sea, I gave myself up to the most voluptuous of feelings, and low and behold from the place where my seed splattered upon the crystal waters rose up the most beautiful of women, naked and enthroned in a scallop shell. She rode on the foam of little wavelets that placed her ever so gently upon the sand. We immediately became great friends and discovered that we had a good deal in common: I, Eros, god of Passion and she, Aphrodite--for such was her name--the goddess of Love. And as you know, we were made it hit-it-off and hit-it-off we did and always have."

Eros initiated Hermes in the pleasures of self-pleasure, as both were careless youths who shared in equal measure life's secrets. Hermes in turn initiated his son Pan.

Pan

God of the wild and shepherds, he has the legs and horns of a goat, as do fauns and satyrs, and because he lives in the wilds--forests, groves and woods--he is connected to fertility. Son of Hermes and a nymph, the mountains of Arcadia were the seat of his worship. Doted with great sexual powers, his phallus is huge, and his father, Hermes, taught him its use through autoeroticism, which Pan then taught to shepherds. While some claim that the Great God Pan died, killed by Christianity, it is only a rumor, and false at that, as Pan shall live on as long as shepherds take pleasure in pleasuring themselves.

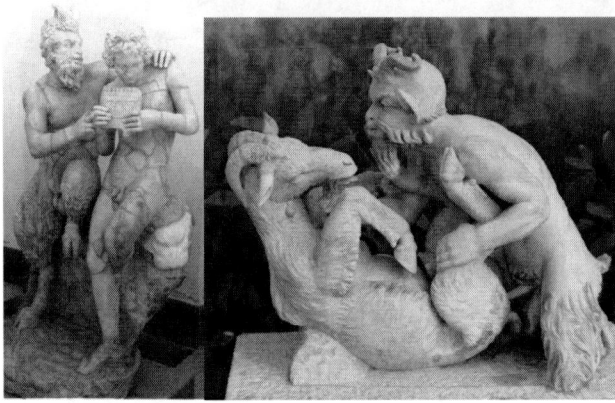

Pan seducing Daphnis and engaging in what some would consider part and parcel to omnisexuality, sex with a beast.

Pan is shown here with his lover Daphnis, a Sicilian shepherd, also a son of Hermes and a nymph. As Pan was himself the son of Hermes, he was committing incest with his half-brother [not counting the persistent rumor that his father Hermes also enjoyed unlimited access to Daphnis' charms]. Omnisexual Pan had fallen in love with the daughter of a river god, her name Syrinx, from which we have our word syringe, who, in order to escape Pan and his ever-erect phallus, changed herself into a reed and hid in her father's river. To have her ever near him, Pan, not knowing exactly which reed was Syrinx, cut several that he fashioned into a flute, a flute he used to attract boys [as seen in the above picture].

A lover of women and boys, incest and onanism, he has become the symbol of omnisexuality.

Daphnis, by the way, also loved girls, one of whom was his childhood playmate Chloe. He now resides on Mount Olympus at the side of his father Hermes.

In Aristophanes' *Ecclesiazusae* he writes:
''It's decreed that the ugly and the wretched get to fuck first.

So take your pleasure on the porch in the meantime, handling your fig-leaves [foreskin] in the courtyard'' [courtyard meaning outside the vagina].

Hippocrates wrote that semen comes from all the body fluids, and is the most important part of them. (6)

Greeks found masturbation a natural remedy to frustration when boys or women were unavailable, just as today's understanding roommate will leave his roomie alone for a few minutes for sole release when he returns from a date, when he declares he didn't get any.

In *The Knights* by Aristophanes Nicias and Demosthenes are going to escape their master, by bolting at top speed. Nicias suggests they start off slowly, ''as if you were masturbating: first slowly, then quick and firmly, at top speed!'' In another play a slave complains that he masturbates so often that his ''foreskin looks like the back of a whipped slave.''

All in all, masturbation was so common in Greece that it was rarely referred to. As in most societies, it was recognized as the domain of boys, and those not getting enough sex with boys or girls or both.

We have this poem by the Greek poet Scythinus, about whom we know nothing:

> Aged 16 Elissus is made for love,
> A wonderful ass as tight as a glove.
> Parted lips, sweeter than honey to kiss,
> A wondrous voice, the sound of bliss.
> ''Don't touch!'' he says, and I'm left to my fate,
> I think of him all night and masturbate.
>
> Erect you are my tall flaming cock,
> Valiant, ready, as hard as a rock.
> When Nemensinos came to my bed,
> You deflated and my face went bright red.
> Now he's gone and you're swollen to the gland,
> You won't get any relief from *my* hand!

Rome

The Roman poet Martial [Marcus Valrius Martialis] wrote: "Ponticus, you never fuck pussy but use your left hand as a mistress, a friend to your lust. But what if everyone did so? There would be no children if we all jacked off and sent our filthy cum into our hands! This is what Nature is telling you: 'What's flowing through your fingers is a human being!' "

Martial also stated that masturbation was an inferior form of sexual release, one resorted to by slaves, although he admitted to it when a beautiful slave-boy was too expense to obtain: "My hand relieved me as a substitute for Ganymede." (5).

Martial also wrote: *"Veneri servit amica manus*, Thy hand serves as the mistress of thy pleasure."

Romans appear to have preferred the use of the left hand, a graffito from Pompeii reads: "When my worries oppress my body, with my left hand I release pent-up fluids."

The etymology of the Latin word *masturbari* is a compound of *turbare*, to agitate, and *mas*, male.

Romans were like Americans in that they were prudish hypocrites. A senator lost his rank when he kissed his wife in public, while human sexuality has rarely exceeded the extent of Roman orgies (9).

CHAPTER THREE

WHAT IS MASTURBATION?
A jerk-off session, how the Ancients did it,
God's and Daddy's gift should include an intact foreskin,
Masturbation versus sports

Masturbation if the manual stimulation of the penis to produce pleasure. From puberty on it usually ends in ejaculation, whereby sperm is expelled through the penis, accompanied by an orgasm, the most powerful and pleasurable sensation the human body can experience. Besides feeling good, it relieves tension, sexual and other, and expulses aging semen in order to make way for newer, more lively and fecund sperm. Boys from age 12 can jerk off 3 or more times a day, with only favorable health consequences.

A jack-off session begins with an erection, the penis often rock-hard thanks to an influx of blood engorging it, an erection caused by erotic thoughts and/or by manual stimulation. It can take place anywhere a boy chooses, although the most comfortable is on one's bed, perhaps rubbing the penis against the sheets [called prone masturbation], but usually ends up with the boy on his back, wrapping your fingers around the penis and moving them up and down, from a full fist if one's penis is long, to several fingers if shorter. In the on-your-back position the sperm, often called jizz, spunk and one's load, bursts out, the body shuddering with pleasure, the pelvic area bucking wildly, the semen ending up on the stomach and/or chest, the flow of which can also simply dribble over the boy's knuckles, or shoot over his head in spurts, 3 to 8 jets, accompanied by a wonderful sensation that can last from 5 to 10 seconds. The semen can be cleaned up with a kleenex, which saves one from embarrassment should a t-shirt or towel, later discovered by one's mom, be chosen.

After orgasms an ''off'' switch kicks in, putting on the brakes, caused by the hormone prolactin. Dopamine pushes a guy to cum at all costs, prolactin makes him roll over and go to sleep, although young guys can often start again in a few minutes, or even straight away.

The anal area has an enormous number of nerve endings that can be stimulated with the tongue or fingers. Women will rarely, if ever, ream a man, but it is a pleasure of untold bliss. The male G-spot is the prostate gland, stimulated by fingers, dildo or a guy's dick, disliked by some men, a pleasure stronger and more powerful than penile orgasms for other men, a pleasure they literally beg for. And don't forget the nipples, hugely erogenous, nor fondling the testicles and the area between the testicles and the anus, the perineum, with special attention to the frenulum with its nerve endings [all explained later], its stimulation ideal under a foreskin if you're lucky enough to have one, with oil or saliva if not.

The Egyptians themselves had a contradictory view of masturbation, just as we do today, accepting it, on the one hand, as normal and even necessary, making it a subject of taboo on the other. Isis condemned her brother Set and her son Horus for engaging in mutual masturbation. As punishment, she cut off her son's offending hand, only to reattach it later, masturbating the boy herself until the wound healed and he was able to take over himself. For Egyptians masturbation represented pleasure, but also pollution, as the waste of semen was the antithesis of creation, because sperm only survives for about two minutes on a lad's belly. During the festival of Min the pharaoh and his followers masturbated into the Nile, as said, an act that otherwise was forbidden in public, in the same way that Diogenes was criticized for masturbating on a street in Athens by the otherwise liberal Greeks. In Sweden a man was recently found innocent of public indecency when he openly masturbated on a beach, although it was clear, at the same time, that such public acts, although perhaps lawful in liberal Sweden, were nonetheless considered disreputable even among Swedes. Of course, everyone masturbates on beaches and in the dunes, obligatory in the sun and fresh sea air, but it's done discreetly, except on gay beaches where it's a key attraction and highly appreciated display of prowess.

Although Hindus, like Lisa Simpson's Buddhists, often denounce sexual pleasure as a cause of human suffering, it was nonetheless the phallic god Shiva who was masturbated by the fire god Agni, who then swallowed his semen, giving birth to Skanda, the god of male beauty, the perfect happy ending.

Chinese Taoism evolved techniques that would prolong masturbation without ejaculation, ejaculation reserved for male-female sexual intercourse, a preference shared by Hindus. The same for Islam, where penis-stretching techniques are used [to be discussed], although in many cases ejaculation is permitted if there are no other means of sex available.

It is true that the hormone prolactin, produced during the sex act, sends a boy into the arms of Morpheus after his orgasm, the proof, according to Taoists, that it weakens the body. And it's true too that if you can work yourself up to near-orgasm and then stop, you do feel a kind of elation, exactly as Taoists and Hindus suggest. [Scientists confirm that by avoiding an orgasm, as sages throughout history have recommended, you avoid the extreme highs brought about by dopamine and the lows of prolactin (see chapter on hormones).]

In Greece masturbation was a natural part of sexuality, a safety valve, depicted on numerous vases. The Greek culture was phallocentric, and statues of the Greek god Hermes were found at crossroads, replete with erect phalli rubbed to a polished luster by boys who sought increased potency, by women who wanted male children, and girls who sought husbands. Their purpose was also to inspire sexual encounters, as crossroads were traditional places where travelers came together. [See my books *Alcibiades* and *Greek Homosexuality*.] Hermes taught his son Pan how to masturbate, and Pan instructed shepherds in the art, the pleasure often shared in mutual orgasms.

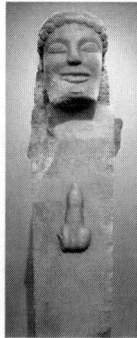

Hermes at crossroads.

Romans accepted masturbation, inventing the word from the latin *masturbari*, meaning to rub or agitate, as well as a panoply of other words, but perhaps because the Empire needed boys as soldiers as well as administrators, the pastime became a gradual defilement, and with reason, in that Sparta itself ceased to exist through lack of warriors, male seed far too often lost between male buttocks (2).

Calamity struck with the advent of Christianity, where saints, themselves masturbators and sexually licentious during their youths, grew into bitter old men who condemned the act and those who did it, while generations of monks and priests, from that time to our own, have used their positions of trust to mislead and defile boys in the thousands, unpunished then, punished today by the simple expedient of the Catholic church paying out *billions* of dollars in damages, but no jail time (3).

Boys can ejaculate in two minutes, and often do it rapidly so as not to be caught. But boys have to learn to slow down, so that they will be capable of making love in real situations once they become sexually active. Studies indicate that if a boy can resist 15-30 minutes without an orgasm through masturbation, he will be able to resist ejaculation during lovemaking for as long as he wants. Reaching several erotic peaks without ejaculating will make for a far stronger final orgasm. And a second orgasm, on the heels of the first, if possible, will often be stronger than the first.

Masturbating in front of a partner shows him/her what turns you on, and in a long-term relationship it has to be admitted because, among other reasons, both people are not necessarily interested in doing the exact same things at the exact same times.

Masturbation reduces stress and releases sexual tension, it helps one become more comfortable with his/her sexuality and erogenous zones, it eliminates the possibility of pregnancy and the transmission of sexual diseases, the reason homosexuals turned to circle jerks before and during the gay plague. It's a cardiovascular workout that lowers blood pressure.

All boys and men masturbate, 55% admit to doing it once a week, 40% daily, and 70% of married men still masturbate regularly, according to one study. A British survey stated that 73% of men had masturbated during the four weeks before their interview, 53% of men during the previous seven days. Gays in relationships masturbate far more than heterosexual men in relationships.

We masturbate because it feels so good. As Woody Allen said, ''It's sex with someone you love'', and there's no reason to not display that someone in a mirror, perhaps while you're showering, a daily visible reminder that you should not skip the gym, and that a little bronzing at the beach or poolside would enhance your beauty, allover if that's how you like it, or in speedos if you like the tanned-body/white-buttocks sexy look.

Nothing will ever replace classical up-and-down hand pumping, pre-cum lubricating the foreskin if, again, you're lucky enough to have one, baby-oil if not. Sex toys can be amusing, hand operated or automatic. Yet, just as the summit of all musical instruments--the piano, violin, flute or what have you--is the human voice, so too are a boy's five fingers his best buddy, from circle jerks to the privacy of the dorm room, where they're hidden in the blankets, well out of the sight of one's unsuspecting roommate, and just the thumb, caressing the frenulum, is enough to admit God and His heavenly choir into the restricted space, now warm and humid thanks to still another glorious spend.

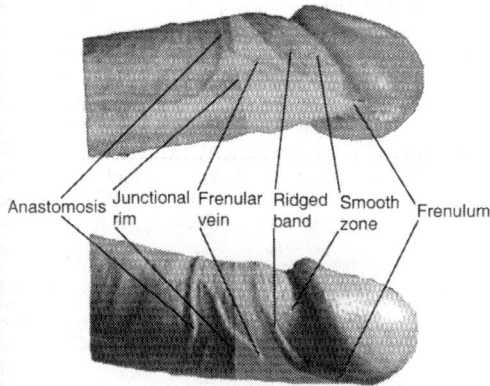

Anastomosis Junctional rim Frenular vein Ridged band Smooth zone Frenulum

The frenulum

Where you masturbate is essential. The ideal location is in bed, where you're warm, comfortable and fully naked, tissues and lube at hand. Taking care of morning wood can be done in the shower, caressed by warm water, soap a great lubricant, even if oils and creams are preferred because they don't dry out the skin, although soap leaves you spotlessly clean. The great outdoors is fine, once you make sure you're unobserved, the beach and beach dunes ideal, the pleasure often doubled because of the ''danger'' that someone just might see you, and if you're gay, there may be participants, a voyeur's dream come true. Jerking off in a car, alone or with a buddy, is great, the best side-by-side masturbation scene was filmed in *El Paso Wrecking Corp*, found, among other sites, on Redtube, at minute 15 of the 46-minute film: https://fr.redtube.com/184804 [the full history of this kind of porn is covered in my book *All-Male Pornography*].

Being naked is the ultimate turn-on, but caressing the head of your levis-clad dick in class, your fingertips gently stroking the stretched denim in circular movements, can be earthshattering, especially because it's in public. Doing it on an airplane john in a matter of seconds, or prolonging it for hours in bed, are alternatives, bringing yourself up, close to orgasm, but not over, again and again, is the basis of tantric sex, even if tantra tries to avoid the loss of semen through ejaculation. The longer you prolong, the more pre-cum--Nature's AAA+++ lubricant--the greater the final result when you eventually give in.

Although we are made in God's image, none of us are nevertheless exactly alike. Some are able to cum in seconds, and then cum again and again, some armed with 9 inches (4), others shooting amounts of jizz that inundate belly and chest, some well over their heads, the majority splatter their stomachs, while a few make it just over their knuckles. The inequality is often abetted by man himself, who perversely deprives us of our God-given right to a foreskin, while we ourselves shave the very symbol of puberty and manhood, our pubic bushes, that which makes us ''all-boy''. Some have fleecy chests to die for, others hairless asses to more than die for. Most are attracted to women, and its boobs that make them hard, others, like the Romans, were attracted by big dicks, those applauded in Roman baths as boys strutted through the corridors, their dicks swaying side to side, the size of which got them dinner invitations at the best Roman tables (5). Whatever sex we may prefer now, the future belongs to omnisexuals, the growing answer to a man's needs [and the norm from the early Greeks right up to the so-called Enlightenment] (1).

Masturbation frees our imagination, one reason it should be practiced as often as possible away from porn books, DVDs and

Internet. It's calming and relaxing, each orgasm proof of our masculinity and sexual power, each of which should be accompanied by a true thanks [to God and your daddy] for our being born with our royal scepters.

Wikipedia sums up things perfectly: The most common masturbation technique, *Wikipedia* informs us, ''is by gripping and sliding the foreskin back and forth and by moving the hand up and down the shaft. This type of stimulation is typically all that is required to achieve orgasm and ejaculation. The speed of the hand motion will vary, although it is common for the speed to increase as ejaculation nears and for it to decrease during the ejaculation itself.'' Perfect. Circumcised males need a lubricant such as spit, which is tragically incomplete compared to Nature's original gift, a foreskin and natural pre-cum.

''Lying face down on a comfortable surface such as a mattress or pillow, the penis can be rubbed against it. This technique may include the use of a simulacrum, or artificial vagina,'' continues *Wikipedia*. ''There are many other variations on male masturbation techniques. Men may also rub or massage the glans, the rim of the glans. Some men place both hands directly on their penis during masturbation, while others may use their free hand to fondle their testicles, nipples, or other parts of their body. The nipples are erogenous zones, and vigorous stimulation of them during masturbation usually causes the penis to become erect more quickly than it would otherwise. Some may keep their hand stationary while pumping into it with pelvic thrusts in order to simulate the motions of sexual intercourse. A few extremely flexible males can reach and stimulate their penis with their tongue or lips, and so perform autofellatio.'' *Wikipedia*, no prude, goes on: ''The prostate gland is one of the organs that contributes fluid to semen. As the prostate is touch-sensitive, some directly stimulate it using a well-lubricated finger or dildo inserted through the anus into the rectum…. Mutual masturbation is a sexual act where two *or more people* stimulate themselves or one another sexually, usually with the hands. It is practiced by people of all sexual orientations, and can be part of a full repertoire of sexual activity. It may be used as foreplay, or as an alternative to sexual penetration. Frequency of masturbation is determined by many factors, e.g., one's resistance to sexual tension, hormone levels influencing sexual arousal, sexual habits, peer influences, health and one's attitude to masturbation formed by culture.'' End of article.

Incredibly, the only truly complete statistics concerning masturbation date from Kinsey, 60 years ago, meaning they are largely meaningless to our Internet generation. Today some boys openly masturbate seated before their computers, careless of the presence of other males, an intimacy unheard of in past generations.

In 2009 the UK joined the Netherlands in encouraging daily masturbation as healthful, mindboggling when one considers the heinous reputation of ''self-abuse'' a few years back, one that continues in most other countries in the world, many of which continue to imprison homosexuals. In a Health Service leaflet in Sheffield entitled *Pleasure* one finds the slogan: *An orgasm a day keeps the doctors away.* It encourages the young to delay losing their virginity, a way of preventing unwanted pregnancies and diseases.

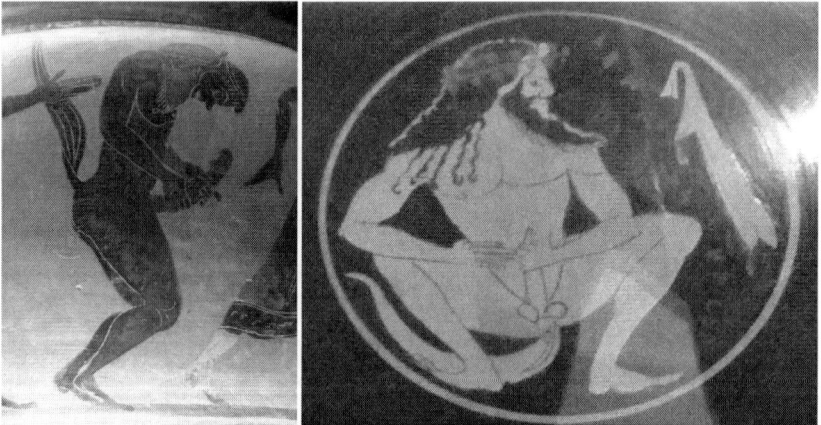

Satyrs – Greek krater – 550 B.C.

Autoeroticism is practiced by married men who generally have to conceal the fact, and by some gays too in a relationship, although gays are far more open to most forms of sex, mutual or alone or shared. It is a pleasant alternative, and as a man never leaves the house without his equipment, it can be performed absolutely anywhere when one feels the urge. In high school and at the university, especially in the library, when aroused, I needed only to move the eraser of my pencil over my buttoned levis fly, hidden by the table, to produce nearly instant ecstasy, *and* release from stress, *and* a welcomed time-out.

A 1997 study reveals that frequent autoeroticism decreases the risk of heart attacks and it seems to lower blood pressure. That said, ''real sex'' is a better cardio-vascular workout, still another study affirms. A 2008 study at Tabriz Medical University states that frequent autoeroticism reduced swollen nasal blood vessels, rendering breathing easier.

In David Bret's *Errol Flynn* we learn that Flynn had a jack-off room in his home that gave onto a bedroom on the ground floor through a one-way mirror in the flooring. He chose the best-looking boys and girls and gave them the use of the bedroom while he and his pals, among them David Niven, bunched around, jerking off while the couples screwed below. Both Niven and Flynn had lives of incredible interest before they'd become stars. Luckily, Niven left us two books he wrote, *The Moon's a Balloon* and *Bring on the Empty Horses,* that are simply wonderful (15).

Diogenes recommended autoeroticism because it was easily available and inexpensive, ''If only one could satisfy one's hunger by rubbing one's stomach!''

For the Hebrews, who needed a big population, autoeroticism was a crime, and for Christianity a graver mortal sin than adultery. Even during the Enlightenment a man's semen was deemed finite, and so autoeroticism was a wasteful loss.

As far as sports go, sex therapist Eric Garrison states that sexual abstinence is superstition, and that athletes tell him they don't want to jinx anything by breaking the pre-game dry spell, no matter how horny. He goes on to say that some of the best professional football, basketball and baseball athletes he'd worked with all wanted permission to have sex before or on the day of a competition, and his advice to them was to go ahead and masturbate or have consensual protected sex. Physical therapist Kosta Kokolis stated that sex before matches was beneficial because it increased blood circulation, improved mood and decreased nervousness. A college player said that ''sex before a game helped relax and gave confidence. It gives you an edge.''

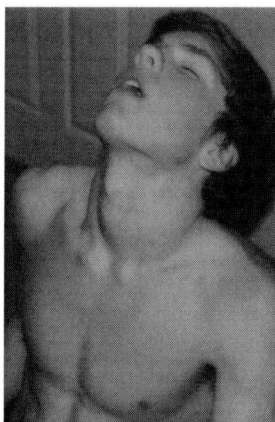

Above all, masturbation is healthy pleasure.
It improves sleep, boosts mood, prevents sexually transmitted diseases, improves heart health, is good practice for sex, increases lifespan and studies suggest it prevents prostate cancer.

CHAPTER FOUR

THE MASTURBATION PANIC
Tissot, Kant, Rousseau, Freud
Circumcision
Berlin
Magnus Hirschfeld, Krafft-Ebing, Christopher Isherwood

There followed the masturbation panic, caused by the beliefs of certain doctors, most notably one whose name has come down to us, Simon-André Tissot, 1728-1797, who claimed that the loss of an ounce of semen equaled the loss of forty ounces of blood, a crippling factor that could lead to the loss of eyesight, to diseases and, due to increased blood flow to the brain, insanity, consequences as damning as religious threats of Hell due to the nefarious, unnatural act of self-pollution, the mortal enemy of procreation. In the mid-1850s masturbation was blamed for the corruption of morals, as well as vile thoughts that threatened the salvation of the soul itself, accompanied by the exhaustion of the entire nervous system. Boys were ordered to do physical exercises until they dropped from fatigue, to take cold showers, and fathers were advised to tie up their sons' hands at night [presumably behind their backs, although the most exquisite sensations could then be enjoyed by gently rubbing oneself against one's mattress, as the reader well knows]. Some surgeons recommended replacing the testicles of masturbators with healthy ones [which could lead to castration because the new testicles were rejected by the body, and death if the surgery was done in unclean surroundings, often the case in those times]. Freud himself showed interest in the possibilities of the operation--for others, not himself.

Tissot was no quack.

He was a recognized and hugely respected scientist and researcher, who studied medicine in Montpellier [home of France's top medical schools], was noted for his treatment of smallpox, awarded the title of First Doctor in 1786 by the King of Poland, a titled conferred the following year by the King of England. Tissot was a Swiss Protestant Calvinist neurologist, physician, professor and Vatican advisor, whose Treatise on Nerves and Nervous Disorders made him, in the opinion of modern doctors, the founder of their profession. Recognized as an authority on migraines, he was acknowledged by Kant and Voltaire, and even Napoleon Bonaparte wrote him, thanking him for ''spending his days in treating humanity'' and noting that ''your reputation has even reached into the mountains of Corsica,'' Napoleon's birthplace.

Kant wrote that masturbation was ''a worse vice than the horror of murdering oneself'' and ''debases the masturbator below the beasts.... It is a violation of duty to oneself.'' [Kant also believed that bastard children were born outside the law, ''stolen into the commonwealth like contraband merchandise,'' and so ''the commonwealth could ignore their annihilation,'' meaning they could be put to death.]

Tissot's 1760 book *L'Onanisme* stated that semen was an "essential oil" that when lost from the body would cause "a perceptible reduction of strength, of memory and even of reason; blurred vision, all the nervous disorders, all types of gout and rheumatism, weakening of the organs of generation, blood in the urine, disturbance of the appetite, headaches and a great number of other disorders." Tissot brings us a concrete example of what he's talking about, concerning one of his patients: " I went to his home; what I found was less a living being than a cadaver lying on straw, thin, pale, exuding a loathsome stench... A pale and watery blood often dripped from his nose, he drooled continually; subject to attacks of diarrhea, he defecated in his bed without noticing it; there was constant flow of semen...Thus sunk below the level of the beast, it was difficult to believe that he had once belonged to the human race." The boy, a clockmaker, had been masturbating three times a day, but, Tissot sort of assures us, "Not all of those who commit themselves to that odious and criminal habit are so cruelly punished, but there are none who aren't afflicted to some degree."

Tissot was far from the only man to scare the bejesus out of boys.

Jean-Jacque Rousseau, Genevan philosopher and writer, wrote to Tissot: "I know that we are made for each other, you and me, for understanding and loving each other. All those who think like us are friends and brother. I am at your feet, Monsieur." And later: "How much would I like, in my last days of sickness, to have Tissot at my side, so that when there is nothing more to be done from the body, he may still be the doctor of the soul."

In his *Encyclopedia* Rousseau wrote that "the only way, according to the views of nature, to empty the superfluous semen, is what nature has established in the intercourse and union with women and its delicious delights. The infamous habit of masturbation, born through indolence and idleness, are forced pleasures that cause an infinite number of serious diseases, which are often fatal." Rousseau wrote that "This vice, which shame and timidity find so convenient, has a particular attraction for lively imagination. It allows them to dispose, so to speak, of the whole female sex at their will, and to make any beauty who tempts them fulfill their pleasure [through masturbation] without the need of first obtaining her consent," the original sin of adultery, committed simply by looking at a person and imagining intercourse with her, "in his heart", as stated in Matthew 5. In his *Confessions* Rousseau nonetheless admitted to lifelong masturbation.

There is no wonder that the boy I was, just entering his teens, who found an old book in the cellar of the grocery store where he worked, was, after reading just a few pages--was, like the eight generations of boys since the death of Tissot, scared shitless.

Circumcision

Why circumcision became the mutilation of a boy's birthright is disputed: some researchers say it was thought to lessen masturbation, a typically American Puritan No-no. Some scientists claim that when the foreskin is not thoroughly cleaned it admits an odor that young boys find pleasurable and draws their attention to their penises, leading to masturbation. Others maintain that foreskins could cause cancer or minor infections if, again, the area was not sufficiently cleansed. Foreskins are thought by some doctors to favor herpes and other sexually transmitted diseases, and in 2014 the U.S. Center for Disease Control and Prevention *endorsed infant male circumcision*, something all medical institutions outside the United States categorically refute. [In Europe it has been admitted that circumcision could reduce urinary track infections by 1%, but this is countered by the number of hemorrhages, infections and even an occasional--if rare--death when a boy is circumcised.]

The Berlin contribution to the Masturbation Panic.

Berlin became the center of sexual research in the 1800s and early 1900s, Magnus Hirschfeld the leader of the pack. The population of Berlin exploded, from the 400,000 in the 1800s to 4 million in 1920. Berlin went from a city of open sewers to the first city ever electrified, with, in 1800, electric streetcars and lighting. It went from a city of open sewers to one of public toilets and baths, from the filthiest to the cleanest city in the world, infinitely more hygienic than London, Paris and N.Y.

Magnus Hirschfeld (1868–1935) was a sexologist who practiced in Berlin. He founded the Scientific Humanitarian Committee with others in 1897, the purpose to promote sexual understanding. His work was inspired by a military officer who committed suicide on the eve of his wedding, preferring death to what would be required on his honeymoon night, an epiphany for Hirschfeld.

Dubbed the Einstein of sex, Hirschfeld opened the Institute for Sexual Research in the liberal Weimar Republic in 1919, that housed a Museum of Sex and had some 50 rooms, one of which was occupied for a time by Christopher Isherwood and visited by W.H. Auden, André Gide and Sergei Eisenstein. There was a museum with sex toys and walls plastered with photos of nudes, presumably there for sexual education, and lots of men dressed as women and women as men, both in photos and live as visitors. Teas were offered at the Institute, reigned over by Hirschfeld and his lover Karl Giese. Bar hopping at night was included, so that in one way or another one could meet and mate with whomever one wished, back "home" at the Institute. For those passing through like Isherwood the occasions to meet boys, the private rooms and stacks of pornography, made the Institute a horny lad's wet dream. [Isherwood's life can be found in my book *American Homosexual Giants*, Isherwood a naturalized American.]

Richard von Krafft-Ebing (1840–1902) was second in importance to Hirschfeld, an extremely influential Austrian psychiatrist, a medico-legal authority on sexual pathology.

The purpose of sexual desire, wrote Krafft-Ebing, was exclusively procreation, "and every other form of sex must be regarded as perverse." Homosexual libido was a moral vice whose origin was early masturbation [and he angered the Catholic church by writing that martyrdom was a form of hysteria and masochism].

Masturbation was held by many as the key to homosexuality, while some researchers claimed--after having examined many men--that active homosexuals had arrow-shaped penises, while their passive counterparts had anuses in the shape of accommodating funnels. Still other physicians found homosexuals to possess small dicks, the reason they were spurned by women who sought out greater sexual satisfaction, and therefore left small-dick guys among themselves: forcing them into homosexuality.

In 1925 Adolf Brand, a German writer and bisexual anarchist (13), wrote that prudent masturbation ''absolutely cannot be harmful. What is worse is to forbid sexual self-satisfaction to young people. A prohibition cannot be kept, since the sexual drive in young people absolutely requires satisfaction. And since the forbidden fruit is doubly enticing, it contributes to the attainment of sexual self-satisfaction. Only under secrecy can self-satisfaction, which is natural and healthy, become a sexual vice.''

Intercourse too was to be restricted to procreation, because if it were practiced too often the result would be the same as for masturbation, the proof being the loss of energy and extreme fatigue after spilling one's seed. This was reinforced by the fact that men in asylums openly masturbated. The final choice was between going to Hell or ending up insane, little wonder the period was known for its masturbation panic. Today things have changed to the extent that a lad is considered a prude if he refrains from jerking off in the presence of a college roommate-- although this has its limits, as we'll see in the chapter on School and Dormitory Masturbation.

What took place in Berlin, sexually between men, was basically tame in comparison to today's backrooms. At the urinals in Berlin clubs, boys flashed their wares, and at tables they allowed johns to put their hands through their pockets, which had been cut away inside to allow seizure of the lads' dicks. Lederhosen was popular in the butch places Isherwood frequented, showing off boys' suntanned thighs. Isherwood was said to have had 500 during the time he was there, from 1929 to

1933. [The full story of Berlin can be found in my book *German Homosexuality*.]

CHAPTER FIVE

SEMEN AND ITS LOSS: ONAN VERSUS MASTURBATION

Semen

The Greek physician and philosopher Galenus [first name either Aelius or Claudius], 129 A.D. – c. 216 A.D.], wrote: ''That fluid is only the most subtle part of all the others, its veins and nerves carry it from the whole body to the testicles. In losing his semen, the man loses this vital spirit too. It is thus not surprising that too frequent coitus weakens, since it deprives the body of what is purest in it.''

In 1604 Dutch scientist Zacharias Janssen invented the telescope and microscope, although it nonetheless took Dutch scientist Antoinie van Leeuwenhoek 70 years to discover, in 1677, ''animalcules'', tadpoles that ''a thousand move in a space as small as a grain of sand'' [that he later calculated at 3 *billion* per grain, although today we know that in one ejaculate there are from 20 to 100 million sperm cells, which in itself is prodigious!]. Leeuwenhoek was duly impressed by what he considered an entire human being in miniature form, the purpose of the uterus reduced to the warm, conducive environment in which it could grow. Some observers even claimed they could make out which tadpoles were male and which were female. Later scientists wondered why so many were deposited in the uterus, when most often only one child came out.

Since the semen of one ejaculate could repopulate the world, the reasoning went, wouldn't the loss of one ejaculate through masturbation be equated with the murder of all humanity? The Pasteur Dutoit-Membrini wrote that to lose one's seed through masturbation was a violation of the law of Nature, the law of God, no less than the annihilation of the system of creation.'' It was both suicide and infanticide. Tissot agreed that it was indeed an act of suicide, the catalyst of a future Apocalypse.

Onan Versus Masturbation

Basically, onanism and masturbation are the same, and have been considered so for generations, both signifying the spending of ones seed outside the vagina.

But whereas masturbation is the manipulation of one's penis for reasons of pure pleasure, the origin of onanism was an act punished by death, the purpose of which was to avoid pregnancy. In Deuteronomy 24 it's written that when brothers live together and one dies before producing a son, his brother will sire a boy on the dead brother's wife, so that his brother's name ''will not be blotted out from Israel.''

Onan had a brother, Er, who was declared evil by God who ordered Er's death. Onan's father commanded him to ''go into your brother Er's wife'' and impregnate her with a son that would be Er's. Onan did ''go into her'' but withdrew at the moment of ejaculation, his seed lost on the ground, punishment for which God took Onan's life. Later it was explained that Onan married his brother's wife for her wealth, yet refused her his seed because he didn't want his heritage to go to a son that would be declared Er's, the reason Onan merited God's wrath.

Opponents of masturbation state that it was the loss of Onan's seed--meant to perpetuate humanity--that riled God, whereas others believe that he died because he refused to obey the word of God, who killed him in revenge.

At any rate, Onan's act is rated as the world's first attempt at contraception.

Basically, any act that takes place outside of the vagina-- fellatio, anal, with beasts, frotting--is proscribed by religious zealots, which include Catholics [for whom it represents lust and selfishness], conservative Rabbis [although Reform Judaism tolerates it or avoids the subject], Moslems and Mormons, while liberal Protestants promote it as a safe alternative to pre-marital sex. [One early Christian text states that just as wine and bread represented the blood and flesh of Christ, so too could one drink semen through fellation, as a kind of fraternal communion, mentioned by Saint Augustine.]

Indian Maharajas believed that sperm became rancid like milk and butter if left to accumulate. They had a woman hired to evacuate the semen within a maximum time of half-an-hour, either by offering herself or by masturbating the Maharaja. The woman was otherwise obliged to remain chaste all her life. This [renewal of semen] took place when it was judged that the Maharaja was not coupling often enough with his wives.

CHAPTER SIX

KINSEY AND HIS REPORT

Kinsey was above all a keen masturbator, an omnisexual who adored watching boys and men ejaculate before him, watching and *participating* in hundreds of solo and mutual masturbation sessions, circles jerks his preference, the reason I will now give him voice in these pages.

Alfred Kinsey is an icon, one whose private life is strange nearly beyond words. Nothing has as yet replaced his sixty-year-old study, and no man has demonstrated his sexual curiosity, so outlandish that he would study the couples he hired to perform sex acts, his nose barely inches from the act itself, missing not a single odor nor sound. He loved to show off in the nude and he never hesitated to corner a fellow researcher, grope him [for Kinsey was basically homosexual], in the hope that the salary Kinsey was paying would convince him to roll over. He told his university students they were free to seek his advice on sexual matters, with the expectation that they would become hot-and-bothered enough then--or later when invited on one of his many camping expeditions--to enter into his favorite sexual pastime, mutual masturbation.

As a young man Alfred Kinsey had it all: Eagle Scout, straight-A student, high-school valedictorian, mature beyond his years, president of his class, of his Biology Club and of his Debate Team, a man they called the Second Darwin, gorgeous in high school, handsome throughout college and, later, Harvard.

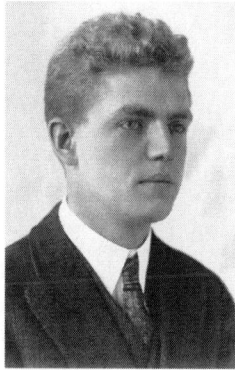

Kinsey always looked more mature than his age.

Lots of high school boys then, around 1912, didn't date, through shyness and slow maturing, while today junior high lads have sex, proof that Kinsey's famous Report, 60 years later, is completely passé. But not Kinsey's life. Photos of Kinsey show him dressed in a suit, as were the other students, a boy who took serious part in the YMCA and Boy Scouts, organizations that were Christian in character, instructing boys against sexual intercourse and masturbation: ''In the body of every boy who has reached his teens, the Creator of the universe has sown a very important fluid. This fluid is the most wonderful material in all the physical world. Some parts of it find their way into the blood, and through the blood give tone to the muscles, power to the brain, and strength to the nerves. His chest depends, his shoulders broaden, his voice changes, his ideals are enlarged. It gives him the capacity for deep feeling, for rich emotion. Pity the boy, therefore, who has wrong ideas of this important function, because they will lower his ideals of life. These organs actually secrete into the blood material that makes a boy manly, strong, and noble. Any habit which a boy has that causes this fluid to be discharged from the body tends to weaken his strength, to make him less able to resist disease.'' [From *Boy Scouts of America: The Official Handbook for Boys*, 1914, brought to us thanks to James Jones in his excellent *Alfred C. Kinsey, a life*, 1997.]

37

Kinsey prayed to God to release him from the terrible vice, that and his homosexuality which, in 1950, was a felony [sodomy and fellatio] in all but two states.

Most boys rationalize their masturbation because, of course, they can't stop themselves from doing it. Lots of other boys, especially in the camps Kinsey was part of, turned masturbation into circle-jerk art, not only jerking off with friends but giving a hand to the person seated to his right. Unlike them, Kinsey felt he had to punish himself, and he did so by pushing an object, at times a straw, down the urethra of his penis and then masturbate. The pain was his punishment, pain that could last for days afterwards.

It was in college, in 1915, that Kinsey apparently admitted to himself that he was homosexual, which manifested itself in his showering and swimming with boys, naked, and fed his voyeurism in the other sports he went out for, especially tennis and golf locker rooms, because Kinsey was an athlete--as well as an accomplished pianist.

He finished college *magna cum laude* and went off to do graduate work at Harvard, in entomology. He received his doctor of science degree from Harvard around 1919 and won the Sheldon Traveling Fellowship of $1,500 [$21,000 today!], thanks to which he traveled through 36 states, 2,500 miles of which was on foot, collecting bugs. He was then taken on as an assistant professor in the Department of Zoology at Indian University in 1920, at age 26.

There, he met the girl he would eventually marry, a near societal obligation in Victorian England, when nearly all homosexuals married (7), one that existed in America too among men who refused to submit to their real sexual preference, men who were sexually confused, men who wanted to be politicians who would never be elected if the truth were known, actors who needed to preserve their popularity among their female fans in order to keep on acting. The pattern was the same: because men didn't seek contact with women it was women who took the lead, imagining that the boy was simply shy, and often after years of basically platonic engagement, they tied the knot. With Kinsey too it was hugs and kisses, and at the time it simply didn't occur to a girl that her beau was a perverted introvert, the lesser of the terms applied to homosexuals--then as now.

Thanks to his girl Kinsey had someone who filled his solitude, who admired him, and who respected his being the perfect gentleman [while in secret he was most probably having "dirty" sex in restrooms and the bushes of parks, or, at the very least, pushing objects up his penis while he had orgasms of semen and blood], and then there was always the possibility that she would cure him of his problem [doctors persuaded actor Anthony Perkins, who let *anybody* have him anally, to marry (a boyish girl had been recommended), and Perkins did finish by producing two children].

The marriage took place in 1921. He later told a friend that no sex had taken place during the honeymoon. He took control over every aspect of his wife's life, and as a university biology teacher his students found him to be arrogant, stubborn, "never giving in for any reason". He fully believed that science could free young minds and wanted his students to be free thinkers, not easy to realize, in reality, when he himself was an unmovable despotic object.

In general he supported marriage as the best way to perpetuate the species and care for the young. The place of his own wife was home caring for him--there was no question of her having a career. He treated her a hair better than the Greeks treated their wives, whose purpose was the care of the home and childrearing, all of which was incredibly strange for the man responsible for two of the world's most gigantically important books. The Kinseys soon had two children, a boy and a girl, the boy tragically dead at age three. Two other children followed, although Kinsey was said to have not been an affectionate father.

Kinsey practiced nudity at home as a way of sex education, and would pull out his member, without pretext, in front of his fellow researchers, a harbinger of later rock stars. He vacationed in nudist camps and participated in orgies, which he revealed in letters to young friends, all men. Masturbation was very often on his mind, and in conversations with male friends he always found a way to bring up the subject, and question them on how and how often they went about doing it. It was not necessarily about research, but a way of finding out if the person would be open to some mutual eroticism. The men who related this, later, had always declined, but how many had agreed, and then kept quiet? He went on field trips, staying in tents, and would spend hours telling the boys around the campfires stories about having sex, the end result was to get them hot enough so that one or several would retire to the discretion behind the canvas flaps. He also spent time in Mexico, where he would warm-up Mexican boys by telling them stories about what he had done with ''hairless'' girls, presumably pre-puberty, all of which put the lads in the mood to ejaculate. His vocabulary was said to have become filthy; verbally and sexually there were no limits. He left word around the campus that if students had questions concerning sex, his door was always open. At the same time he decried the lack of research concerning sex, all of which was the catalyst for the future that would turn his tawdry lifestyle and attempts at sex with anyone at any cost, into his worldwide reputation as a scientific genius. Just like the German Magnus Hirschfeld who was known for his years of sexual research in Germany, an occasion for Hirschfeld to fulfill his own sexual desires, and Baden-Powell, the inventor of the Boy Scouts so close to the heart of Kinsey, yet a man reported to have had sex with an incalculable number of boys, in South Africa and India, so too was Kinsey on the road to limitless orgasms, with ''subjects'' chosen from a population of hundreds. The difference was that Kinsey also had a scientific side to him, one that has made his work, many believe, faultless in precision. [We should perhaps judge a man by his contributions to the advancement of his fellow men, and not his private life: Sir Laurence Olivier, whose private life would make some cringe (17), and who had used his fame and position to entice lads onto his casting coach, nonetheless produced and starred in *Hamlet*--so do we really need to know that went on backstage? Such is our conundrum with Alfred Kinsey, a man who ordered his wife home while he partied with all the enthusiasm of a Messalina.]

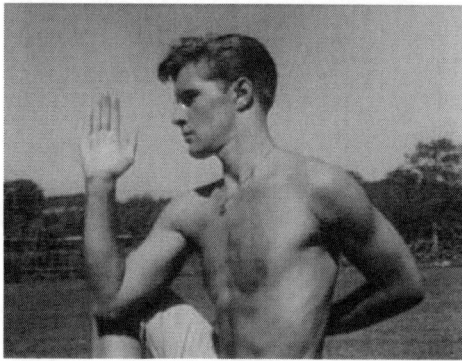

William Miller, intimate with Kinsey and Somerset Maugham.

Several hang-ups have always been part and parcel of an American's life, perhaps the inner belief in Calvinist hard work that could be jinxed by too much sexual felicity. During my years in Rome I was amazed at the ease with which Italians accepted their sexuality. I saw boys parade around their homes and have breakfast in their briefs, *served* by doting mothers and sisters, while at the beach young lads would pull down their swim suits to compare fully-erect phalluses and pubic bush growth, the adults around them sleeping like sated seals. In reality, American sexual beliefs were still dominated by Victorian ideals, and that into the 1960s (7).

Kinsey had had a lifetime of unanswered questions, and the more he interviewed his students, the more he discovered the scope of their, and his, ignorance. Doctors who should have led the way to enlightenment hammered nail after nail in the coffin of sex, providing lists of the mortal diseases whose roots sprang from self-abuse, doctors who labeled homosexuals as hermaphrodites, perversions that Nature had embodied with both sexes.

The more Kinsey delved into the subject of sex, in small groups that soon developed into full conferences, the more he decided to do something about his and his students' ignorance on the subject. He was one of the first to take an interest in endocrinology, and became convinced that there was a male sex hormone that would be the answer to all outstanding questions. [In 1889 a Harvard professor injected himself with an elixir derived from dog testicles. He felt more vigorous, but abandoned his research due to the criticism of fellow professors. Two scientists received the Nobel Prize of 1939 for isolating testosterone, and its vital role in sex became clearer in the 1950s and '60s, years after Kinsey had predicted the existence of the hormone.]

In 1937 Kinsey gave a lecture in which he introduced a slide showing a real vagina being penetrated by a real phallus, and told the students exactly what was going on pleasure-wise [going so far as to tell the boys to use spit as a lubricant--boys who probably hadn't as yet discovered that saliva was great in simply jerking off]. He certainly had the boys' dry-throated attention, their dicks just as certainly rock-hard, as this was the first vagina and the first fully-deployed phallus they had ever seen, outside of their own.

By 1938 Kinsey was no longer handsome, but thanks to his classes and conferences he no longer had to go looking for people for sex. People now pursued him, an earth-shattering difference in the life of a man set on having a maximum number of orgasms [as would, much later, pornstar Al Parker (12)]. The more he freed his students from their sexual ignorance, the more they opened up their minds and bodies to him, all of which makes me wonder if Hugh Hefner ever had it so good?

In 1939 he went on the first of many trips to Chicago to visit the gay community that was anonymously established in big cities to escape attention. He appears to have taken great care of the gays and was probably sincere in the friendships he formed, as his letters to the boys there demonstrated true fondness for them. He invited several to his home in Indiana to meet his family, all of whom he treated with great respect. His weak spot, one present in many homosexuals, was his difficulty in accepting effeminate boys whose effeminacy, he told them, was learned, and so advised them to un-learn it. It's true that many homosexuals desperately want to be men in the image of heterosexual men, and so have little tolerance for those who lack outward virility.

Sexually, Kinsey took advantage of his outings in Chicago, certainly blowing and being blown, certainly sauna sex, perhaps glory-hole interludes and anal intercourse [all of which are integral part of his research notes], and like all the homosexuals he frequented he could spend the night slumming and the next day act as if, when he came across the men of the evening before, he hadn't received their semen in some intimate part of his body.

Back on campus student interest in his classes and research had grown to the point that two fraternities told him that 100% of their members would enter into his program. Thanks to his knowledge and fatherly ways with boys, he would woo, what?, some?/many?/most? into his bed, drawn by their beauty while they, as with Alcibiades and his liaison with the homely Socrates, were drawn to his experience and erudition (6).

In my book *Secret Societies* I go into the history of the Bloomsbury Set, where sex of unbelievable dimension was going on, in which some girls would mate with boys simply because the boys were the lovers of the men the girls really loved, and sleeping with the boys was a way of getting nearer to their true loves. It has been suggested that Kinsey's wife slept with the boys Kinsey slept with, as a way too of getting closer to her husband. At any rate, he passed her around to whoever took her fancy. He didn't care, and probably never had cared.

As his university courses were found not exactly "proper" by an increasingly larger number of faculty members, deeply jealous of the crowds that filled his classes and conferences, he took his research off campus. There are a huge number of foundations in America, and several came to his aid, the king of the mountain being the Rockefeller Foundation. Kinsey had to meet many of its people to get his research funded, but as he had already collected a whopping 8,500 sexual histories [his proclaimed goal being 100,000], the needed money was forthcoming.

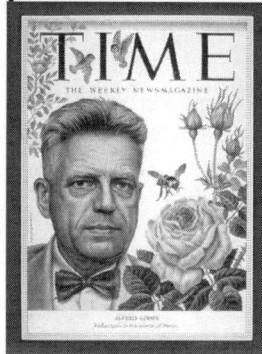

Time 1953

He hired interviewers, all sexually experienced, and when told by several that they were occasionally "attacked" by the interviewees, Kinsey told them to be passive, showing neither interest nor disdain, and he turned out to be right--there was apparently nothing that cooled ardor more than passivity. The men he hired were not exempt from his trying to have sex with them. One fled, confessing years later what Kinsey had blatantly tried to do to him--disgusting in the sense that the men had the choice of surrendering or losing their jobs.

Kinsey encouraged sex among the researchers themselves and regularly attended sexual encounters between his interviewees, and often watched people in action, his face inches from what was going on. Sexually he was insatiable. Photos were taken and films were made, and Kinsey assured one and all, on film, that all sexual problems could be surpassed with patience, desire and vaseline.

"Kinsey considered religion the source of most human misery," writes James Jones. "He had not the slightest doubt that religion was the root cause of sexual repression.'

Early on in his research Kinsey discovered that boys who did not finish school had the most orgasms, while college boys had the fewest. Working-class boys had orgasms through intercourse, college boys had most through masturbation.

When his research came to an end, he had no problem finding an editor as they had been following his work for years and wanted a chance to capitalize on it. In fact, the competition became cutthroat, with everyone trying to lean on those they knew inside the Rockefeller Foundation, to get the sought-after grail. The book hit the stands in 1948, and all hell broke out.

200,000 hardback copies sold in just two months, at $6.50 [$65 today!] for 804 pages. Nothing leaked out concerning his homosexuality and, indeed, he was congratulated on the "ideal" 30-year-long marriage he had with his wife. Margaret Mead criticized him for his serious, puritanical stand, for nowhere did he state that sex was "fun". If the gal only knew! Amidst the euphoria of his success the Rockefeller Foundation accorded him $40,000 to continue his good works.

I read the book years later, far too late to help me confront my adolescent hang-ups, but the case studies fueled a huge number of orgasms, as did the drawings of naked cave men, at the time, in *National Geographic* magazines, nothing sexually visible, of course, but it was all the world could offer in pornography then, and for me it was plenty.

A book of that nature caused huge discord in scientific circles, which apparently weighed heavily on Kinsey as everyone who knew him found him exhausted and all said he'd aged well beyond his years. James Jones compared him to the mainspring of a watch that was wound tighter and tighter. At the same time, flush with money, he enlarged his research team for the express purpose of increasing the number of his sexual partners. Sex between them all became an unsaid obligation if they wished to remain. It was like Andy Warhol's Factory (9) where everyone was forced to participate in the orgies. One researcher did stress that Kinsey was *also* having sex with women.

In 1948 Kinsey decided he would like to see exactly how men climaxed in masturbation. He hired a 17-year-old hustler, an extremely beautiful boy, to organize a session that would involve 2,000 men. The line of participants, each receiving $2, wound down the street and around the block, and although they didn't get the 2,000, they did film hundreds of orgasms [sheets were placed on the floor of the room where the "research" took place, and replaced when soaked through]. The "beautiful boy" had come through with lots of very young beauties, for which he was paid $2 a head. [At around the same time Pier Paolo Pasolini was recorded as having lined up 25 boys on a beach outside Rome--the beach where he was later murdered--and jerked off each one, considered the ultimate in eroticism by those who hadn't heard of Kinsey's doings.]

By the way, the session did prove that most men's sperm did not shoot out as seen in porn films, but rather "dribbled" over their fists.

Kinsey had many contacts with homosexuals who were stressed out of their minds by their "dirty" conduct. He assured them that they had nothing to feel guilty about, and to those trying to become "normal", he told them that it was as easy for a heterosexual to become homosexual as a homosexual to become heterosexual. Meaning: Don't even try.

As said at the beginning of this chapter, Kinsey was noted for being stubborn, and thanks to the incredible success of his book his stubbornness was reinforced, and his way of handling Foundation members who sought information concerning the reliability of his statistics [statistics put in question by scientists everywhere] was not always gentle, although he did usually try, at first, an amiable approach, often inviting Foundation members to his home for dinner. How much Foundation trustees knew about what went on in Kinsey's research center between the researchers, or how he employed underage lads to procure other underage lads for mass sessions in masturbation, is not known. What is known is that the Foundation men, for the most part, were Christian family fathers, who would certainly have put the brakes on if they'd had an inkling of the no-holds-barred acts Kinsey was filming. Opposition came from groups that disputed Kinsey's statistics, scientists who thought he had bent the outcome of his interviews to support the results Kinsey himself wished to obtain. In truth, Kinsey had to battle hard against a huge array of opponents, but he did so brilliantly, proof being that the Foundation continued to fund him, even if the stress greatly harmed him physically.

He was convinced that he was brilliant, and that his research was valid, but no matter how extraordinary he found himself, I wonder if he could have imagined that, 60 years after the publication of *Sexual Behavior in the Human Male,* his name would still be familiar to every educated household in the world?

Yet he lived in an inner hell, one described in excruciating detail by James Jones, when Kinsey, unable to inflict enough pain on himself through introducing objects into his urethra, tied one end of a rope around his testicles, the other around an overhead pipe, climbed on a chair, and then jumped off.

Kinsey's book, and the book that followed on female sexuality, caused so much unrest and dispute that funding dried up, and he spent what remained of his time on earth chasing nickels and dimes to keep his research center open, and for the first time he charged fees for his conferences.

He traveled to Rome where only the sexual underground interested him, and the only monument that caught his attention was the Coliseum, at night, where sex took place, one of many sites favored by Gore Vidal [who knew and contributed to Kinsey's research] (10). He went to Portugal where he complained about not getting laid as often as he wished. Back home he went on with his research, until felled by a heart attack in 1956.

It could have been such a marvelous life. Like all the men who are great in my eyes, he used life and allowed life to use him, the very meaning of our existence. He had his research and the backing of his researchers, all faithful and accepting of his ways. Yet his inner demons pushed him to desecrate himself and his body, as T.E. Lawrence had done (7), Lawrence who should have died by a bullet in Damascus, before allowing himself to be whipped mercilessly by boys Lawrence paid to inflict the pain, and Kinsey should have died directly after the publication of the work that makes him famous to this day, before stringing himself up by his balls.

CHAPTER SEVEN
EROGENOUS ZONES
The brain, ears, mouth, nipples, six-pack, shaft, scrotum, anus
HORMONES
Testosterone, Dopamine, Prolactin, Serotonin, Oxytocin

EROGENOUS ZONES

Every man's body is different in terms of its sensitivity to touch, and the only way to find out what turns it on is through exploration. Although a lot of boys learn how to exploit the sensitivity of their dicks thanks to friends who show them how, an amazing number seem to make the discovery by themselves, through the handling of their instruments when pissing or when washing during a shower--they touch it, it feels good, and one things just leads to another. Some men, although rare, ignore the pleasure offered by their manhood unto their first sex act, which was the case of Rich Merritt who subsequently became a pornstar, his life recounted in a separate chapter.

Boys don't have to know that the area of greatest penile pleasure is situated at the glans and the frenulum, because that's the place they naturally grip when pulling to orgasm.

THE BRAIN

The male brain--thanks to millions of years of evolution, the aim being the survival and continuation of the species--is hardwired to seek out sex. It is the center of emotions, the Polaris of hormones and nerve endings, the neurochemical cocktails the brain dispatches throughout the body, the site where our life experiences lead us unerringly in the direction of whatever makes us as hard. It's the site of our fantasies, the weathervane of how we feel about ourselves and others.

Studies that compare the male and female brain in situations of sex are highly inconclusive, which is just as well because I have no intention of these kinds of comparisons, although I'll immediately break the rule with this disclosure: a man's lust-lever surges at the site of videos showing nudity, heterosexuals before female nudes, homosexuals when viewing naked men, while females apparently show an equal interest in both sexes, leading one researcher to maintain that all females are basically bisexual, a subject gone into in my book *Omnisexuality*. Nor will I enter into the specifics of which parts of the brain are responsible for this or that sexual response, other than to point out that it's the hypothalamus that's associated with male sexual arousal and penile responses to sexual stimuli.

Along with lust, the brain sends out inhibiting messages that keep men from behaving inappropriately, but these are temporarily deactivated as orgasm approaches, ''robbing us of the voice of reason'', as one study puts it. It's unrestrained lust that makes men menacing if their sexual *élan* is interrupted, that drive them to pullover, after dropping off a squeamish bitch, and jerk off, the understanding of which motivates his college roomie

48

to accord him some undisturbed time when he returns from a date, frustrated.

THE EARS

The ears are ranked with the scrotum by some men in sensitivity, apparently more so as orgasm is reached, and in frotting and mutual masturbation a few well-placed dirty words can help bring a guy up and over.

THE MOUTH

The mouth, associated with deep tongue kissing, is a primal booster of dopamine, the lust hormone, and it releases oxytocin, called the love chemical because it helps in bonding with one's sexual partner, the reason some men really do love the person they're dallying with, even if, when it's over, they couldn't get rid of him/her fast enough. The lips themselves are packed with nerve endings.

NIPPLES

Nipples are the unsung heroes of male sexual pleasure. The nipples have one function, gentlemen: to provide us with erotic felicity. In that they are comparable to a woman's clitoris, the only body organ dedicated to sexual pleasure, and just the manipulation of the nipples can bring some men to orgasm. Neurologists maintain that there are 3,000 to 6,000 ultra-touch-sensitive nerve endings in men's nipples, to which they add 2,000 to 4,000 erogenous nerve endings, both groups intertwined, we're told. The glans has 8,000 nerve endings, the clitoris 8,000 and, get this, the foreskin 20,000. So those who tell you that circumcised dicks are as sensitive as the uncut variety, are feeding you bullshit.

Nipples get wonderfully hard during sex [and in cold weather], really baby dicks in their own right, made to be licked, nibbled, sucked and manipulated with the fingers, while stroking one's shaft.

One nipple is always more sensitive than the other, a sensitivity that can be destroyed by piercing, which, by the way, takes 4 to 6 months to heal in that area.

The nipples are part of the pectorals, that men adore to sport, notably to other men who are capable of appreciating the work that goes into their building and upkeep.

THE SIX-PACK

Descending from the nipples and prior to the pubic bush is an area begging to be kissed and licked, its navel included. Guys love to show it off, especially in the locker room, and love to see it in the privacy of their showers, in the bathroom mirror. It and firm buttocks are the centers of attention in locker rooms, appreciated by men of both sexual preferences [although for perhaps different reasons].

THE SHAFT

The penis is the mechanism through which we climax, improved and accelerated when the stroking is done in tandem with manipulation of the nipples. Although comparable in nerve endings with the clitoris, the comparison stops there because men have a secret weapon, testosterone levels far higher than women's, which push us to levels of randiness that women could never dream of, the life-giving elixir that make boys the crazy, often fearless little bastards we are.

The penis shaft is by far the biggest part of the penis, and has the fewest nerve endings. But the bigger it is--the longer and thicker--the better it feels under one's hand, which can be a challenge in oral and anal sex. Ways to make it look its longest, thickest and horniest, especially when soft in a school gym and locker-room setting, can be found in my book *Phallus*.

SCROTUM

The scrotum is highly sensitive, and cupping it with the hand as orgasm approaches can make a guy sigh with pleasure, as well as foreplay in which the balls are licked and, if the sack is loose enough, each individually sucked.

ANUS

The anus is ''rich in nerve cells'', the closest my research has allowed me to get to an actual number, and licking and tonguing it, along with deep tongue-tip thrusts, is an indescribable pleasure to all men, although largely unknown to heterosexuals because women will only rarely, if ever, go there. It has gays whimpering with ecstasy, the more so as tongue trusts are deep and repeated, the partner doing them knowing that his turn is coming up. Even when women try, they lack real enthusiasm, in the same way that in order to be well jacked off a guy needs the healthy, full-strength grip that only a male can bring to another male, not the skinny bicep-reduced arm of a girl.

Entering the anus with a finger or fingers may hit the male P-spot, the prostate, at times sufficiently to produce an orgasm without even touching the shaft, the receiver begging for harder, deeper and faster, so powerful the body shudders with pleasure. It's use in sex has been linked to improved prostate health, of no mean importance as a guy ages.

HORMONES

TESTOSTERONE

Testosterone is what makes us men. It empowers us, and that from a boy's earliest years, making even a 9-year-old so inexplicably wild that his parents can only chalk it up to boys-being-boys. If a 9-year-old's testosterone level were equivalent to a cup of beer, during his teens it would explode to his imbibing 2 gallons a day! It's the magic potion that gives us our muscle mass, bone density, deep voices, body hair, growth spurts, dick size [length and girth] and our yearning to use it until we're both worn out [and our body odor, as well as, alas, acne]. It's what pushes us to leave waitresses unfathomably huge tips, the reason Vegas casinos deck theirs out in the skimpiest of wear.

A study of 4,000 men showed that those with high testosterone levels were 50% less likely to marry, 43% more likely to divorce and 38% most likely to have extramarital affairs. For those who marry, many have a lifetime to regret their decision, once they realize the fleeting nature of beauty--the reason so many men marry when young, when they're dumb and full of cum, as they're the first to admit [after it's too late].

Porn vastly increases the levels of testosterone by 35%, hugely augmenting sexual arousal, as well as decreasing exhaustion.

[Older men may be able to compensate for decreasing levels of testosterone through injections, and some studies even infer that the lower the level of testosterone, the greater the risk of prostate cancer. Low levels are also cause for memory loss and dementia of the Alzheimer's type, believe some researchers. Whatever a man decides to do in this domain must *obligatorily* follow serious consultations with a medical expert--not someone who will give you whatever you want because you're able to pay him for it, knowing that you will return to have the prescription refilled again and again.]

DOPAMINE

Dopamine is dubbed the motivation molecule, and is behind drives, from sexual to sports to daily activities, producing ''excitement, enjoyment and even euphoria'', claims one sources, the lack of which leads to demotivation, lethargy and depression. It's produced through exercise, sex, watching porn, shopping, gambling, computer games, smoking, foods like bananas [a magic source of vitality], avocados, sugar, fatty foods, ice cream and caffeine, cold showers, cannabis, and there's a 400% increase when taking cocaine and a 200% increase through nicotine [as well as 1000% from amphetamines]. Doctors warn that one should get one's dopamine from ''habits that benefit rather than harm you.''

Dopamine encourages promiscuity and invites us to move on to a new partner in order to create greater genetic variety. Rising and falling levels of dopamine are comparable to a roller-coast ride, driving us from depression to recklessness, from lustful sex to making intolerable demands on one's partner.

PROLACTIN

Prolactin kicks in after orgasm, an off switch of such magnitude that a man wants to roll off his partner and roll over into the position most comfortable for his sudden and irrepressible need for sleep. The honeymoon is over when the dopamine level of one partner rises while the prolactin level of the other is high, one wanting sex, the other not at all.

In orgies dopamine pushes a guy to cum at all costs, prolactin makes go to sleep, as said, giving the next guy in line his chance. The woman is still ready for more, an assurance that she'll end up being fertilized by the most valiant and hardy of the semen she receives, as it's believed that only the strongest of men's sperm will be first to hit the target (9). Prolactin is responsible for depression, depending on its levels, creating highs and lows in a relationship, with the possible loss of one's sense of wellbeing.

SEROTONIN

Serotonin is called the happy molecule that puts one in a positive mood. Low levels are linked with depression. It is found in dark chocolate, green tea, cold-water fatty fish, yoghurts and sun bathing, while alcohol and caffeine lower its levels.

OXYTOCIN

Oxytocin is called the love hormone, said to play a role in creating bonds in relationships, such as increased love, loyalty and trustworthiness. Its highest levels come with sex, massages and exercise. This kind of trust sometimes opens girls to the wrong guys, bad boys they believe can best protect them, resulting in many a broken heart.

CHAPTER EIGHT

SCHOOL AND DORMATORY MASTURBATION
Oxford, Cambridge, J.A. Symonds, fagging, Princeton Rub, ship berths, Healthystrokes
Real-Life Sex versus Masturbation

In tandem with the mediocrity of an education in both Oxford and Cambridge, was the poor physical condition of the writers, poets and other aesthetes, of the 1800s and early 1900s, that frequented both schools. Yet they were convinced of their excellence, even if many were nothing but arrogant wimps, often moneyed, who paid for rent-boys in pre-W.W. II Germany and Italy, an easy task in those years where a lad would sell himself for the proverbial Hersey Bar [after the war most boys sold themselves for even less because they were *starving*]. Many Oxbridge boys didn't see war because physically unfit to be recruited, poor eyesight, bird-breasted chests, precocious varicose-veins, girlish biceps. The exceptions were spectacular: Rupert Brooke, Byron and several others, yet even Byron was only attractive when illness brought his weight down to human levels. Few of the men from Oxford and Cambridge resembled the boys seen in gymnasiums or on the wrestling mats, although the boys they paid for were often physically splendid. Proud of the clothes they donned for extravagant meals and the robes they wore in the inner chambers of their rooms, coquettish and swishy, they wouldn't have turned on even a girl, let alone far more demanding males--effeminate twits that make England the last place virile males seek out their own, although there are, and have always been, remarkable exceptions. Writer Wyndham Lewis called Duncan Grant ''a little fairy-like individual who would have received no attention in any country except England'' (11), which, in a nutshell, is exactly what I'm talking about, the reason why the English themselves look to other lands for good sex. [Although for me personally, Duncan Grant was gorgeous, and his paintings marvelous.]

Professors and students took sherry together and shared meals, after which what naturally happened when young men wished to please their masters did happen, consisting most probably of little more than mutual masturbation, but when it took place one time it was hard to see how the inexperienced student could [or would dare to] ward off a second and then a third occasion, and so on, which meant, in the end, that it was a disgraceful debasement of what should have been a striving towards academic excellence. It was putrid exploitation. In the Greek way the lover served as a tutor, whose quest was to academically instruct the boy as well as sexually share acts of love, but the difference was that the Greek boy always chose the man, and that the man was but a few years older, handsome thanks to boys being physically trained, from childhood, to care for their bodies, whereas in Cambridge and Oxford the tutors were flabby, pale-skinned, often androgynous wrecks. We know nothing of Byron's sexual encounters with his tutors, although they most certainly took place, but we do know he had the consolation of lads younger than he, for whom his experience, eloquence, fine clothes, wealth, title and tastes made him a god, a god who willingly released them from their virginity if they had managed to keep it till then, which, knowing boarding schools that catered to lads 12 and over, was highly improbable (7).

About his own schooling, John Addington Symonds wrote: ''The talk in the dormitories and studies was of the grossest character, with repulsive scenes of onanism, mutual masturbation and obscene orgies of naked boys in bed together. There was no refinement, just animal lust.'' The first order that Makepeace Thackeray received on his first day at school from a schoolmate was ''Come & frig me,'' he later wrote.

Dormitories were no more than male brothels. To make sex easy and accessible, [a healthy boy being able to ejaculate six times daily], the linings of their pockets were cut away so they could play with themselves, even in class, and two boys could especially practice mutual masturbation, withdrawing their hands from the other's pocket in a second if interrupted. For unknown reasons homosexuality was more fashionable in some schools than others, and even in schools where it was fashionable it suddenly ceased being so, whereas where it was little practiced it might come back with a bang. In one school a headmaster who succeeded in rounding up a huge number of boys, said to have been around 100, and having them all beaten for some forgotten rascality, was applauded by the boys afterwards for having been clever enough to catch them all (7).

Sex between boys is easy because boys are carbon copies of each other. They know exactly what to do sexually. This rarely goes beyond sexual discovery and experimentation in countries that do not have boarding schools because societal pressures literally push boys into the arms of girls. But in British dormitories what followed sexual discovery was years of sexual intimacy, with only minor exploration with girls that a lad could pay for, and only those with a serious heterosexual bent chose to pay for what they could get for free each night thanks to their roommates. What was easy among themselves became far more complicated on that unknown continent which was women. Everything, there, had to be learned anew, and psychologists maintain that boys who have not known girls from the very start of their sexuality will never experience the fullness of love, the intensity of orgasm, that they knew nightly with boys. Public college boys who married were rarely fully sexually content, and either they had boys on the side or they depended heavily on masturbatory skills.

Fagging was traditional in boarding schools until the 1970s and 1980s. It consisted simply of new, young boys acting as personal servants to senior boys, and was supposedly invented for the purpose of teaching the young lads how to be of service, while being disciplined and receiving instruction from the senior. The lads cleaned up after the older boys, did chores for them, prepared breakfast and teas, polished shoes and ran errands, and spared them the need of exertion by masturbating them to climax, if ordered. What happened sexually varied enormously from one prep school to another--running the spectrum of testosterone-fueled orgies to nothing-happened-at-all [according to some]. Seniors didn't need to revert to actually raping the boys, but as they had supreme power over them in the form of social status, age and physical prowess [captains of various sports were most often chosen as Fag Masters, rarely boys of intellectual ability], the boys had little choice, meaning that even in cases where the youths did not want their anuses invaded they submitted anyway, which of course was a form of rape. This did not stop the same youths from offering themselves to those they liked or loved, in the sanctity of their own dormitories.

The Princeton Rub

The Princeton Rub is also called the Ivy League Rub, a form of mutual masturbation which is highly enjoyable because the nerve endings of the frenulum just under the glans are stimulated through friction, while the participants are in a position to kiss, in the knowledge that there is no risk at all of the transmission of disease, all the while relieving sexual pressure, a physiological need imposed on the body by millions of years of evolution, the aim being the reproduction of the species, even if, in this case, that aspect is sidestepped. Indeed, other primates like the bonobos regularly have recourse to what is also called frottage, cock rub, sword-fighting, the Princeton-First-Year and the Oxford Style or Oxford Rub. It is an alternative to anal sex and is commonly available to boys who may prefer the warm, enjoyable welcome of the vagina, but without the bother, expense and time needed to convince women to let them take their pleasure. Between males no explanation and no financial expenditures are required, just blissful discharge of accumulated semen.

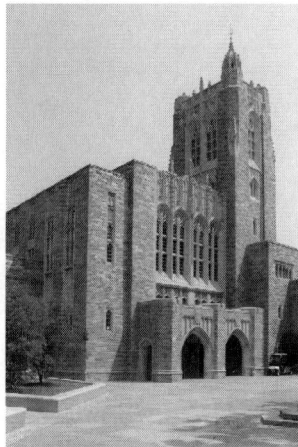

GG-rubbing [genital-to-genital] was popular in Oxford and Cambridge during the last two centuries too, with a great deal of mutual masturbation, less fellatio, but more anal intercourse, as *young* buttocks have been considered more penis-accommodating than those of older men, a belief held since the early Greeks.

Those wishing to encourage phallus-to-phallus sex maintain that it is mutual in the sense that one boy is not ''passive'' [effeminate and degraded], a bottom to the more virile male who is the top. No matter how one wishes to dismiss it, a bottom will always be feminized, the reason why many boys who love anal sex insist on flip-flopping, one cuming in his partner, and then the partner cuming in him. Friction against the prostate is said to offer intense pleasure to some boys, and even *some* heterosexual rent-boys love being fucked for this reason when their johns insist on anal penetration. As in vaginal intercourse, nothing will replace anal sex as the most intimate way possible of becoming close to one's partner. Anal sex--the ultimate step following mutual masturbation, frottage, fellatio and rimming--is becoming more prevalent today thanks to Internet, which shows boys exactly how it's done and the intense pleasure it can procure (4).

Masturbation frequency among undergrads

A majority of undergraduates said they masturbate at least once a week.

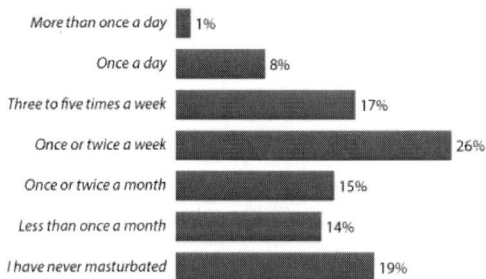

More than once a day	1%
Once a day	8%
Three to five times a week	17%
Once or twice a week	26%
Once or twice a month	15%
Less than once a month	14%
I have never masturbated	19%

Ship Berths

Ships have traditionally served two functions, boys' schools and boys' dormitories. Off the ship a lad's uniform was the envy of boys tied to the land, their pockets always had a few coppers, the women were plentiful and cheap, and as lads always, *always* drank, taverns were even more plentiful, and if one didn't want a girl, one was always certain to find a mate who would welcome him, especially if he paid for a round of drinks. The flipside was when a man wanted to marry and settle down. How could he amass enough money to establish himself? He couldn't hide it in his cot, especially as ships were known to sink. Who on land could he entrust it to, and how would he recuperate even a farthing if he were shanghaied, as was the case when a ship needed new bodies? In addition to this inconvenience, there were far more accidents on a ship than experienced by a servant serving his master tea; there was exposure to the elements, sickness and disease, as well as wars, storms and shipwrecks. But it was life, an incontestable chunk of real life.

Men on ships had long trousers they could role up, and short-waisted jackets worn over heavy kitted jerseys--a wool garment that originated on the island of Jersey--that kept them warm. Due to contacts with Polynesia, tattoos had become popular, even among the most educated classes like that of Joseph Banks on Cook's voyage, although Banks himself hid his on his buttocks. Those who had tattoos, weather-beaten faces and hands scarred by rope burns, were visible targets for pressgangs. The men on ships were given an average of eight pints of beer and rum per day which helped them face their strenuous work, the alcohol content of which they burned off rapidly. Shore leave took place regularly, allowing the men access to drink and women, for a price. Women were also occasionally allowed on board if the men declared them to be ''their wives'' to officers stationed at the gangplanks. The expression ''shake a leg'' comes from the fact that early in the morning men were awoken to begin the day's work, while women sleeping overnight could avoid being roused by shaking a feminine leg outside the covers so that the officers, seeing they were not sailors, would allow them to sleep on. A good captain made sure his men had lemon juice against scurvy, as well as meat, alcohol and hard bread, vegetables and fruit when available.

What took place aboard, sexually, was basically mutual masturbation, intercrural sex [between the legs] and anal intercourse. Fellatio was far less referred to during trials, on sea or on land, likely due to extremely poor hygiene. Fellatio seems to have been part of upper-class sex, certainly due to more frequent baths or perfumes, although bath-taking then was in no way comparable to our own nearly fetish need to smell good.

During voyages there were often long hours of doing nothing, and so one passed the time with tobacco and drinking and occasional mutual satisfaction, usually shared masturbation, mostly on ships but also on land. Even when one paid for the favors of, say, a young drummer boy, the cost was a quarter, compared to $3 for a woman. One man on a ship said that during his entire career he never met a single man who hadn't had sex afloat.

Healthystrokes.Com
[Referred to as HS in this text]

HealthStrokes.com is a Net site that offers excellent advice to, basically, high school and college students. What surprised me most was something HS wrote about how uncomplicated sex is in high schools, in comparison to colleges and universities. I personally went to a Mormon high school in Salt Lake City where I'd never even heard the words fuck and shit uttered orally, not in the locker room, not even at the University of Utah where some Mormon kids dared drink coffee in public. Sex was a forbidden subject and kids married virgin. I clearly remember my very best friend cursing a guy too interested in my friend's girl, sputtering that if the guy were that uptight [horny being another forbidden adjective] he should go home and jerk off. I'd never heard ''jerk off'' stated out loud either, and it made me turn beet red. So when HS declared that today high school boys not only joke about jerking off, they do it at times together, especially during contests to see who could shoot the farthest and the fastest, I was amazed. On the other hand, apparently, *college boys* skirt the subject of masturbation, seemingly as shameful at Utahns. HS suggests that roommates pin up their class schedules so that each knows when the other will be out of the room, allowing each to find relief in private, carefully emphasizing that the word masturbation need never be used when the suggestion of mutually posted schedules is brought up. The key, for HS, is to arrange private times for each roommate. Neither has to specify what the private time is used for, the very mention of the word seemingly [and surprisingly to me] highly embarrassing. Otherwise, ''as a rule, guys just wait to masturbate until their roomie is asleep,'' states HS.

Because one masturbates on the sly, masturbation becomes less frequent than in high school, to the point that some college students even start having nocturnal emissions for the first time in their lives. HS maintains that boys who live in single-sex dorms are less sexually active than those who live in co-ed dorms, who themselves are less sexually active than guys who live off campus, which is of course far more expensive than dorms. It's a situation especially ridiculous when one considers that campus stress could be hugely alleviated through the comfort of a daily orgasm. High school boys jerk off up to several times a day, college lads far less, although HS states that guys screwing girls nonetheless jerk off 4 times a week, while sexually inactive boys do so once a day. ''College boys who have sex the most [with girls] also masturbate the most.''

HS gives its seal of approval to the Homer Simpson method: Hang a necktie over the doorknob if he's with a girl, or a sock if he's with a picture of a girl.

Good communication between roommates can exist, to the point that when a roomie returns from a date, complaining that he didn't get any, the roommate may choose that moment to take a shower, giving his friend time to relieve date-pent-up frustration. Some heterosexuals can have friendly enough relations with their roommates so they can sleep naked, if such is their preference [it sure as hell was mine at that age], and even share the same girlie magazines, jerking off in private or in the presence of the other, lights out, and in a couple of emails to HS boys mentioned jerking off with his roomie while watching porno, or doing it separately in bed, lights on, although I imagine that this may depend, in part, on the boys' omnisexuality (1). Sex discussions can be so taboo that two gays could share a room for a year without even suspecting the sexual bent of the other. If a boy like Matthew Burdette [in the memory of whom I end this book] can commit suicide simply because he was caught masturbating, imagine the consequences for a boy exposed as being homosexual.

''This guy was so cool,'' wrote one college student about his roommate ''that he gave me his schedule so I knew exactly when I was going to be alone in the room.''

One of the boys, age 19, wrote HS that he was jerking off in a shower stall and sort of ''shrieked'' when he came. When leaving the stall, a guy in another stall looked at him questioningly. ''The water just went cold!'' said the boy.

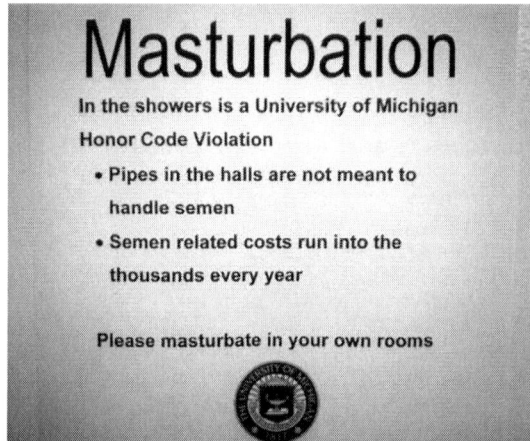

Masturbation

In the showers is a University of Michigan Honor Code Violation

- Pipes in the halls are not meant to handle semen
- Semen related costs run into the thousands every year

Please masturbate in your own rooms

One guy said he'd masturbated only twice in the dorm during the 4 years he was there, but made up for it weekends at home, 5-7 times.

On the other end of the spectrum, several guys complained about their roommates who openly and unselfconsciously masturbated. HS suggested that the offended roommates ask the offenders to please do it in private, not an easy task in our Net culture. The proof is a video showing a kid jerking off in front of his computer and then making cackling noises like a chicken when his roommate leaves the room. The boys in the video are young enough to be high school students, which perhaps underscores the reality of sex being easier and more accepted then than later in college.

Another lad wrote that he and his roommate masturbated when the other was in class. They then talked openly about sex and wound up having jerk-off sessions together, without ever touching. One got married, the other his best man.

One highly amusing email was sent by a boy of 13, worried about being obliged to jerk off in front of delinquents and their guards if he were sent to a reformatory. The advice HS gave the lad was to stay out of trouble, because, if he were ever sent to a reformatory, jerking off publicly would be the least of his problems.

Another guy, whose strategic thinking will certainly make him a candidate for the CIA, wrote that not being discovered jerking off was a way of keeping others from going after his girlfriend: ''If they know I'm jerking off they'll think I'm not having sex with my girl, which will open the door for them to give her what I'm not.''

A final example of HS advice: ''Refusing to talk to your roommate about privacy issues [which need not mention masturbation specifically] does nothing to keep him from knowing that you masturbate but keeps you from enjoying it fully.'' And: ''Arranging to have privacy in the room is key.''

Real-Life Sex versus Masturbation

The subject above concerns masturbation, a lot of which takes place when a guy comes to his room after a date, his dick rock-hard because he didn't get off.

So the question of how much ''real sex'' is taking place in colleges comes up. The answer is, plenty.

LifeStyles Condoms has done some very serious studies in sex, the following taken from a recent Sexual Satisfaction Survey, involving students aged 18-24.

All had had sex:
33% several times per week
12% several times per day
18% every few months

Concerning the number of partners they'd had so far:

86% had from 1 to 10, of whom 38% had between 2 and 4,
10% more than 15.
44% wore condoms most of the time
23% rarely or never

Concerning fidelity:
44% were in a serious relationship
42% had casual sex
78% of the serious relationship group said they never
cheated, although 22% said they would if they knew they
wouldn't be caught.

As for how it's done:
32% prefer the girl on top
28% the boy on top [missionary]
25% doggy

Does size count?
83% of the girls like to be hammered by big dicks
Nearly all the boys wanted to be bigger
[My book *Phallus* goes into the incredible lengths boys go to
to look bigger, especially heterosexuals who want to look their
sexiest and longest, when soft, in a locker room with other guys!

CHAPTER NINE

WHERE TO MASTURBATE, OILS AND TOYS
Computer comfort, gay Paree urinals, circle jerks, the Beggar's
Benison, Jacks Clubs, soggy biscuits
Oils and Toys
Phone Sex
Cyber-Sex

Computer Comfort

Having sex seated in front of one's computer is the absence
of fear of failure, cringing at remaining soft while a girl's waiting

to be serviced. In Net pleasuring a boy is concentrated exclusively on himself, and he can become hard or soft or take a break, his orgasm when *he* wants it. Watching porn begins before puberty because one can't go to the Net without fortuitously falling on a sex site, which leads to masturbation before a boy can cum, as he simply does what the other boys on the screen are doing, the eventual result his first spending, around age 12. Because what one sees on the screen is often more erotic than real-life sex, because it's far more stressless, sex with girls decreases once a boy has gotten over the excitation of his first physical contact with a vagina, once the novelty of ''real sex'' with a girl has worn off, once it has become mundane, and mundane intercourse takes its place among all the other means of getting-off, the very definition of omnisexuality (1). Boys discover that sex among themselves is the simplest way of fulfilling the need to share warmth with another human being because there is zero obligation, because both are united for human comfort and the sharing of a mutual ejaculation, where in heterosexual intercourse the girl expects satisfaction and the boy knows his role is to supply it, plus the after-service, taking her to a restaurant, concert or what-have-you.

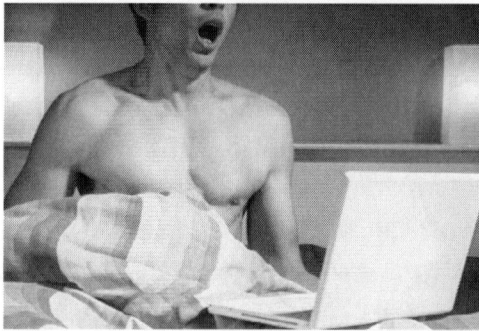

Computer sex is an orgasm when *he* wants it.

Some sources claim that the phenomenon of ''over masturbation'' exists, but whether it exists or not, self-pleasuring does diminish a boy's lust when he meets up with a girl, after having already satisfied himself, perhaps multiple times, and lacks the randiness known to pre-Net boys who found themselves in a car at night with a girl that their bodies were screaming to impregnate. Married women are the real victims of Net pornography, as not only have their husbands grown accustomed to their bodies following years of usage, but how could they possibly compete with the girls just 18 that men see on their computer screens, their breasts siliconized melons? Interviews with married men reveal that many can only climax with their wives by replaying porn images in their mind's eye, while most other men take advantage of their wife's absence to jerk off seated before what one man called ''my other woman, my computer.'' As I fully explain in my book *Phallus*, during sexual stimulation two hormones, dopamine and oxytocin, are produced, both responsible for sexual pleasure, sexual addiction and sexual bonding, all of which is transferred to pornographic images via one's computer, the new inamorata.

Gay Paree

The centers where masturbation was practiced changed after George-Eugène Haussman destroyed the myriad of streets and alleys in favor of today's large Parisian boulevards, work started in 1854. Before Haussman the streets were less lighted, the alleys so dark a man couldn't see his hand before his face. They were ideal arteries for robbers, and in the morning the dead--from brawls, murders and thefts--were collected for burial in common pits [thrown into the Seine in earlier times]. Sexually the narrow streets were paradise, where any alcove, cul-de-sac, doorway and arcade sufficed for a rapid exchange of mutual orgasms. The parks where men met were the same as under Louis XIV, headed by the Tuileries and Palais Royal, but during the Belle Époque these two were largely replaced by the Invadiles, the Champ de Mars, the gardens of the Luxembourg, Parc Manceau and the Champs-Elysees with it trees and bushes and urinals, supplemented by bars, restaurants, cafés and baths, massage parlors and discrete male brothels (21). Heterosexual whorehouses also catered to those clients looking for boys, sending out for a lad who didn't mind sodomizing a man when the price was right. Urinals were a Parisian singularity, 4,000 in 1904 [!], where mutual masturbation took place in the twinkle of an eye. At the time there existed even cubicles where men could piss without being spied on, but these soon became glory holes so popular that even when the holes men drilled were sealed with cement, even when they were welded shut, they were back in use a week later, the purpose masturbation and fellations.

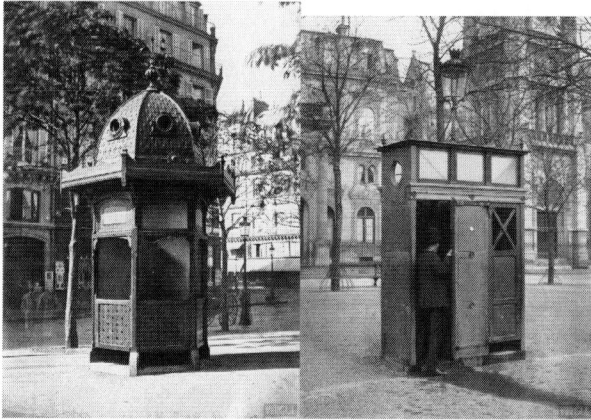

Examples of individual urinals.

L'École Militare, Les Invalides and the Champs de Mars were popular for those in search of uniforms because military barracks were housed there, as well as the seat of military government [many an afternoon I waited, seated on the low wall around Les Invalides, for my own soldier boy, Laurent, at the end of his duty, who would approach with a smile, perhaps for me, perhaps for the gift I invariably brought for him (14)]. There were military barracks at the Vincennes woods too, which made it popular, and the Bois de Boulogne was coming into vogue, the center today of mass orgies, women in cars, naked under fur coats they open when they've parked, the car doors locked, fingering themselves while hordes of boys look on and ejaculate over nearly every inch of the women's Jags, Mercedes or BMWs. Gays have their fun more deeply in the forest.

It was amazing the time the police spent in trying to find someone guilty of ''*outrage public à la pudeur*'', public offenses against decency, because otherwise they could do nothing in a country that had no laws against homosexual activity, whereas across the Channel in Britain any form of gay sex was punished by fines and imprisonment [and death until 1861] (7). In America gays were being trapped in Central Park, until the Stonewall Riots of 1969 (19).

Circle Jerks

As boys are obsessed by their genitals, they have made the circle jerk an erotic form of art, the pleasant memory of which is part of nearly every heterosexual's boyhood.

A circle-jerk is typically defined as ''a group of men or boys forming a circle to masturbate themselves or each other,'' though it has come to mean any form of mutual masturbation among three or more people. About his own experience one boy wrote: ''The 'circle jerk' is one of my first memories. We all stood around in a circle, told stories about girls and rubbed our penises until we got hard-ons. Then we ejaculated. The purpose was to see who could ejaculate the farthest.''

The Beggar's Benison

The Beggar's Benison was founded in 1732 in the small town of Anstruther in Firth of Forth, comprised of men of all ages and social ranks, to celebrate the conviviality of male sexuality and free love. The men ''frigged'' upon a Test Platter, at times as many as a score. The Test Platter had an engraving that showed an erect penis and vulva.

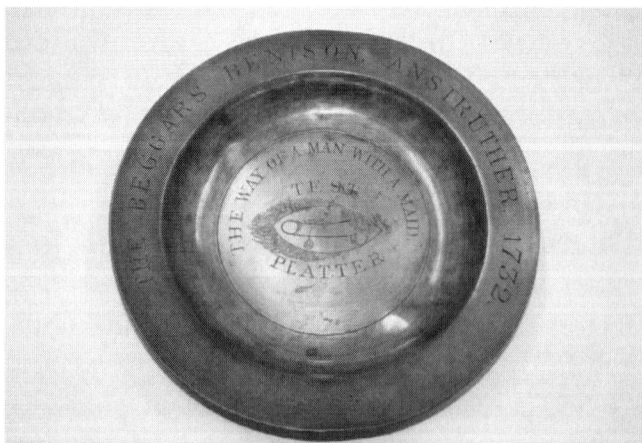

New members ejaculated over it while older members came up and placed their members against that of the new boy, an erotic welcome.

The Benison was founded during the Enlightenment, in opposition to the Puritan view that sex should be reserved for procreation within marriage, a proclamation that sex was pleasurable in itself. As usual in Victorian England, women were placed on a pedestal, exactly where men wanted them, freeing men to find pleasure elsewhere [the number of male and female whorehouses exploded during Queen Victoria's reign, the showplace of omnisexuality (1)].

At the Benison, girls were employed to excite the men, aged 15 to 17, masked, paid for, that the men could observe close-up but apparently not touch. The masturbation sessions came later, when the men were among themselves.

Benison meant ''blessing,'' and the club's motto was, ''May prick nor purse [one's money] fail you.'' The men dined, drank, sang bawdy songs and made lewd toasts.

The Test Platter was covered with a white napkin over which the new boy, called a novice, placed his erect penis while, two by two, older members came up and touched the erect penis with their own erect phallus.

The Benison kept a record, an example of which is this 1737 entry: ''On St. Andrew's Day, 24 met, 3 tested and enrolled. All frigged. Two nymphs [young girls] 18 and 19, exhibited. *Fanny Hill* was read. Broke up at 3 o'clock a.m.''

It closed shop definitively in 1836.

Jacks Clubs

The San Francisco Jacks

The San Francisco Jacks was founded in 1983 as a reaction to the gay plague, and continues to this day, inspiring Circle-Jerk Clubs in all major cities, even in my hometown of S.L.C. The mission of all Circle-Jerk Clubs is to promote comradery through jerking off in the presence of others, singly but usually mutually, oral and anal sex forbidden. At the San Francisco Jacks attendance is around 60, aged 30 to 65, and the men bring their own beer, while lube and paper towels are provided. The absence of youth and good-lookers lessens the sexually stimulating aspects of the goings-on, which leaves the comradery and shared human presence. A witness to one of the bi-monthly affairs stated that everyone ejaculated at least once. With the discovery that fellations were relatively safe, and the awareness that rubbers can be sexy, most encounters now take place in the traditional clubs, saunas, parks and docks that existed before the plague.

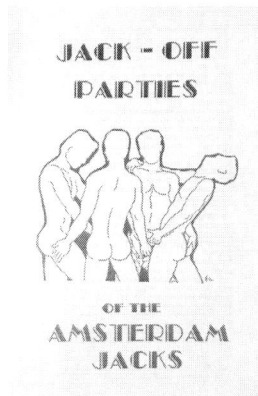

JACK - OFF PARTIES

OF THE AMSTERDAM JACKS

The Amsterdam branch of Jacks

Seattle Rain City Jacks

A "provincial" kind of Jacks gives one a differing point of view, although the Seattle Rain City Jacks is one of the oldest and longest lasting of jack-off clubs. Around 60 men meet at a time, at the origin simply a place where men liked the congeniality of being with other men, but like most jack-off clubs, it got a boost when the gay plague took on epidemic proportions. The specificity of the Rain City Jacks is that its membership has remained high, and it has the record in the number of events it's hosted, 300, since the early 1990s. Many of the participants are bi, some are exploring their sexuality, and an amazing number are thought to be heterosexual, there for male-bonding, who consider sex with men as "recreational penis play." This particular club charges $25 a year. Some members wear wrist bands, red meaning "Don't touch my dick'', green ''Touch without asking'', and no band, ''Please ask first.'' The furniture is said to be comfortable [although canvas-tarp covered (!)], and oil and paper towels *à volonté.* The lighting is dim, the music soft and without female voices. The showers are stocked with skin-care stuff.

''Younger guys still associate fucking with conquest, with rites of passage, with achievement of adulthood,'' states a participant, the reason condom-sex is back in saunas, backrooms and bathhouses, so most jack-off clubs have gone the way of the dinosaurs. In jack-off clubs there is little competition, the atmosphere relaxed and content. But then, these guys are rarely the stunning bucks found in an Amsterdam sauna, whom everyone competes for.

In general, jack-off clubs started up in the '70s, the outgrowth of private parties, but with the gay plague entire lofts had to be hired to take in the capacity crowds, and just like in Ancient Rome (5), guys who have 7'' and over are applauded. Unlike saunas, where the most prized boys are hasted off into private rooms, in jack-off clubs everyone is allowed to do some stroking on premium dicks, or at least some furtive touching, and palming a mammoth member, even for a few seconds, can make a guy's night.

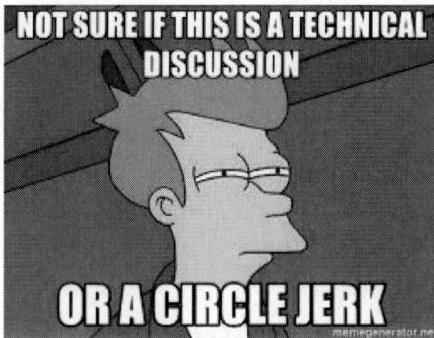

NOT SURE IF THIS IS A TECHNICAL DISCUSSION OR A CIRCLE JERK

The New York Jacks

The New York Jacks was formed in 1980. The early groops had two mottos, ''No lips below the hips'' and ''Nothing goes inside anybody's anything", meaning there's a lot of touching, kissing and nipple nurturing.

Soggy Biscuits

It's impossible to know how often the circle jerk known as the Soggy Biscuit takes place. I would say rarely, but the reference to it in many sources bespeaks otherwise. Boys ejaculate over a biscuit, the last to cum obliged to eat it. In Australia it's called the Soggy Sao, named after a square Australian biscuit. One source claims it's a common practice in the Australian Navy.

It's actually shown in the 2013 film *Wetlands*, a whole group of boys around what appears to be a pizza.

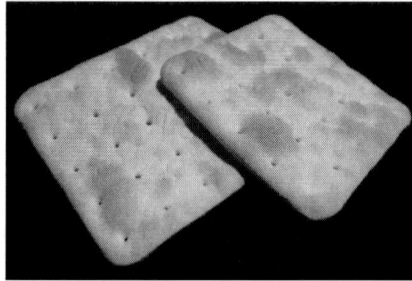

Sao Biscuits

Manhood Camping Firequest

This was published on Craigslist, an American classified advertisements website:

Manhood Camping Firequest. Lookin' for a 100% for real bros to share/experience manhood in all its glory. This is for real, I don't want to waste my time or yours. 100% JO and manhood, no sugar added. I AM NOT GAY. Don't even think this is a sex thing, it's all about manhood.

Looking for bros to head into the woods and bond by fire, experience life as men once lived it, JO circle, and fire/vision quests.

THIS IS NOT A SEX THING.

Gonna need some basic things/skills, I don't want to be slowed down by fools:

- must be in reasonable shape, if you get winded walking then stay home
- Ed Hardy camping gear, it's really good gear and it's awesome
- desire to be a man among men
- not afraid to wield a blade
- crystal, I'm not sharing mine

- must be able to make a fire
- gloves
- a knowledge of native vegetation (knowledge of psychotropic fungus a plus)
- knowledge of modern music
- protective/splash resistant eye wear
- 5 - 10 of those clip things that rock climbers use

We are gonna need a mobile music device, ipod or something. I'm bringing the music for the firequests and visionquests, Nickleback's The Long Road. I only have it on CD, so I'll have my discman as a last resort, an ipod would be nicer. Just sayin'.

Dont' want to see"

- bad attitudes
- gay/homoerotic behavior, this is a manhood thing. I AM NOT GAY.
- cock rings, can't keep it up w/o help, you aren't gonna make it on this quest
- firearms, there's gonna be enough guns going off and spent shells to pick up
- the nerds/dorks/lames/and anyone less than 100% into manhood.

If you are serious, then I promise you this will be the trip of your life. It will change the way you think. I'm serious, and I AM NOT GAY. To see a group of bros being men, a JO circle by a camp fire. The charge/energy in the air. You will slip into a different frame of mind, you will feel electric.

Last outing, we had a group that was so charged we attracted bears. It was no deal, nature knew man was in the forest, the crystals [drugs] gave us the confidence to own those bears. I saw it, I was there.

100% SERIOUS, NO FAKERS

Craigslist Poster Seeks Partners For "Manhood Camping," Totally Non-Sexual Group Masturbation

Oils and Toys

Some guys like to jerk off using lubrication, others don't bother. Your dad gave you your engine, and if he was intelligent and carrying, he left you your foreskin, a huge boon in giving yourself pleasure because, among other benefits, there is no, or little, lubrication needed. If you were mutilated through circumcision, oils, hand creams and saliva are fine, and soap is great during a shower, although it can enter the piss-hole and sting, and also, claim some, dry out the skin. Water-based lubes are recommended, these said to be among the best: Climax Bursts, Mood Warming, Gun Oil H2O and Smooth and Slick, and this Silicon-based lube that doesn't dry out ''and can take a pounding'': Pjur Body Glide. [Man1Man Oil has spent a fortune advertising its product, a ''medical'' approach to penile skin moisturizing, so it won't be ''dry and dull-looking'', as well as treating the ''micro tears'' that ''allow bacteria to penetrate'',

73

leading to "infection." Man1Man will repair raw and chaffed skin, cracks caused by "too much masturbation", as well as acne and folliculitis, the inflammation of pubic-hair follicles (both of which I was too dumb to know even existed as threats to the penis). The cream "restores reduced sensitivity", and helps with discoloration of the penis (?), "as well as bending and curving" (!?!?). The Man1Man ad goes on for *pages*.]

Male sex toys are used, among others: PDX Elite, Head Honcho and Optimale Endurance Trainer Ultraskyn Stroker, although the top two are said to be Fleshlight and Kiiroo. New electronic masturbators come with video inscriptions, the porno film sending out messages to the machine that will reproduce what's going on in the film, sucking in a man deeply, for example, when on the screen the male performer plunges to the limit. The idea is that men take their pornography *personally*, putting themselves in the place of the man doing the action.

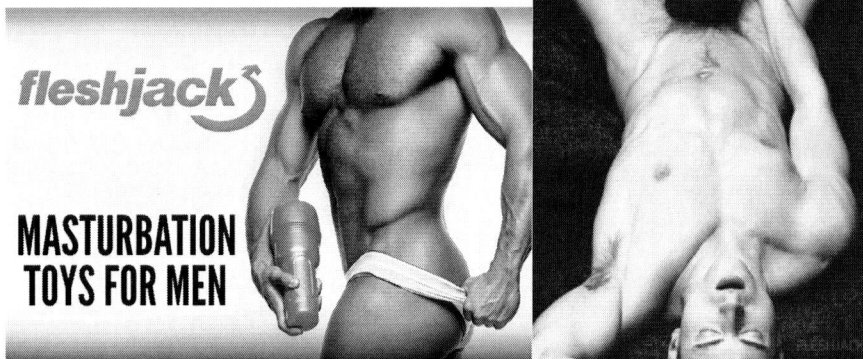

The conventional fleshlight, $50-$100, and look at the size of the new toys, around $200.

The most popular sex toy today is the smart phone. Apple has just come out with a new larger version, after believing for years that smart phones would be too cumbersome to ever become big, underrating a boy's need for the biggest images possible when he jerks off in the school john or the nearby mall.

Phone Sex

Phone sex began with phone companies themselves billing per-minute, part of the proceeds going back to the number dialed. In this case the woman [in hetero sex calls] would try to keep the man caller on the line the longest time possible before his orgasm. Pressure by right-thinking women put an end to this, so that a caller would thereafter have to pass through a private provider, giving his credit card number and pre-paying for a specific length of time: 10, 30, 60 minutes. The provider then relayed the caller to the home phone of the kind of woman he wanted, black, college, etc. [called phone sex operators, fantasy artists, adult phone entertainers and audio erotic performers]. In this case the man was encouraged to climax rapidly, using up, say, 20 of the 30 minutes he'd paid for. He lost 10 minutes, which permitted the girl to take another caller 10 minutes faster, while being paid for the full 30. In 2002 phone sex earned an estimated $1 billion, phone companies receiving $500,000. Durex claims that in 2009 45% of the UK population had used phone sex lines. In 2013 there were over 2,000 phone sex companies in Britain, many of the sex workers female university students.

Cyber-Sex

Text-based cyber-sex has been in practice for decades, and consists of sending sexually-explicit messages. Webcam sex consists of two-way video connections during which the person on each side of the connection performs sexually, usually accompanied by dirty talk. Cyber-sex can be recorded and diffused on the Net. It has been the basis of successful adultery suits, and is considered a form of infidelity by many. Commercial webcam sites allow people to have sex while others watch them and masturbate, in exchange for money. There is no safer way of sexual gratification, and because it's done in real time, with real-time verbal exchanges, it can be highly erotic. Five popular hookup sites are FriendFinders-X.com, AdultFriendFinder.com, Passion.com, GetItOn.com and iHookup which reportedly has

216,000 new members monthly at a monthly cost of $39.99. These sites are dedicated to masturbation, and represent a new way, among many others, of getting off, from *Top Gun* toilet sex to mom and dad missionary.

CHAPTER TEN

MAJOR EVENTS TIMELINE
Montaigne, Diogenes, Kant, male chastity belts, Wilhelm Reich, Thomas Szasz, Philip Roth, Michel Tournier, Joycelyn Elders, Harvard Medical Research, Graham and his crackers, Kellogg and his corn flakes, sperm banks, Matthew Burdette

1576 – Michel Eyquem de Montaigne invented the word masturbation when he wrote this concerning Diogenes: ''For Diogenes, practicing masturbation in public was expressing the wish, before by-standers, that he could satiate his belly by rubbing it.'' Montaigne continues: ''When asked why he masturbated in the middle of the street, Diogenes replied, because I am hungry in the middle of the street,'' a personal freedom Montaigne defended as long as it is done ''in moderation and without interfering with the freedom of others.''

1600s – In the Puritan colony of New Haven, Connecticut, ''blasphemers, homosexuals and masturbators'' were eligible for the death penalty.

1743 – Robert James, an English physician, wrote *A Medicinal Dictionary* in which he described masturbation as being ''productive of the most deplorable and generally incurable disorders'' and wrote that ''there is perhaps no sin productive of so many hideous consequences.'' James invented a quack powder for the cure of fevers, a bestseller at the time.

1797 – Immanuel Kant, philosopher, labeled masturbation as ''a violation of one's duty to himself'' in his *The Metaphysics of Morals*, adding: ''a man gives up his personality when he uses himself merely as a means for the gratification of an animal drive."

1829 – Sylvester Graham was a Protestant, a frail and sickly boy obsessed with health, convinced of the dissolute power of sex. He rose through the ranks of his church, telling his followers that meat brought out their animal instincts. "Wholesome food made wholesome people," he said during services, earning him enemies who stormed his lectures, butchers and bakers, the first responsible for the sale of meat, the second for making products from white, highly refined wheat. He also counted men among his enemies who were offended that he would discuss sexual matters in the presence of women.

Graham decided to produce a food from the king of nutriments, unrefined wheat, stating that the refined, white, version made for "a lazy colon." The product had to be bland, in opposition to foods that stimulated sex: meat, coffee, spices and alcohol, as well as anything sweet, as sweets have always been held responsible for sexual excess, just as chocolate is considered, today, an aphrodisiac. The resultant graham cracker, brittle, was perfect for school boxes and camping trips. Buyers didn't find it all that bland, because it became a huge success, and has remained so for nearly 200 years.

1838 – Jean-Étienne Esquirol, a French psychiatrist, wrote that masturbation was the "recognized cause of insanity in all countries."

1856 – 1932: Between these dates the U.S. Patent Office awarded 33 patents to inventors of anti-masturbation devices: Leather, and leather and steel corsets, metal penis tubes, spike-lined penis rings.

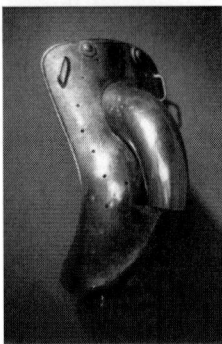

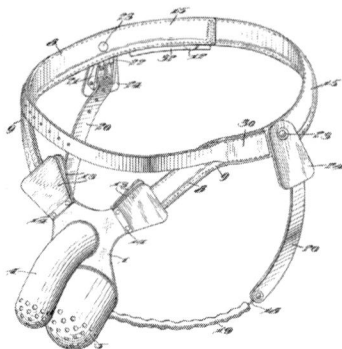

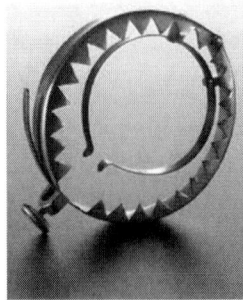

1880 – Cereal magnate John Harvey Kellogg invented Corn Flakes, a bowl of which would create a spirit of morning goodness that would--when accompanied by regular cleansing of the bowels through enemas--dispel any ideas youngsters had of self-pollution. Kellogg, a doctor, nutritionist, "health freak" and shrewd businessman, declared that sex for anything other than reproduction was "sexual excess" [and the cause of acne]. Like many others, he felt that the caressing effect of foreskins, which led inevitably to self-abuse, could be cured by removal of the foreskin itself through circumcision.

1884 – Professor William Pancoast of Philadelphia's Jefferson Medical College performed the first artificial insemination resulting in the birth of a child. The first sperm bank opened in America in 1952. Today mostly boys 18-45 are recruited as donors. Men's production rooms are provided in the UK, a masturbatorium in the U.S., where they masturbate into a collection condom, with the aid of pornography, such as videos, magazines, photographs, both sexes represented. The first commercial bank opened in 1971 in Minnesota, from 1990 in the UK.

1922 – Wilhelm Reich worked in a Vienna clinic associated with sexually-related problems, especially the role of masturbation, and revealed his finds in a paper he presented to the Vienna Psychoanalytic Society. The paper stated that there were three categories of male masturbation, the first having the male masturbate against sheets and pillows, an improvised vulva, orgasm at the end of rhythmic thrusts of the pelvis. This indicated a strong inclination towards the opposite sex, which Reich found healthy. The second was using one's hands, the most common form, which was autoerotic and acceptable. The third was in front of a mirror while reading rape scenes, or in toilets, public parks or mutually with friends, done by those who were mentally disturbed.

Reich himself is of such interest that I'd like to go into his life: William [Wilhelm] Reich [1897 – 1957], worked closely with Freud. His name was yelled out by students during the May '68 Student Revolt in Paris because he encouraged coeducation, with the sexes allowed to mingle and have intercourse when they desired to do so. In his diaries he told of trying to have sex with the family maid with whom he slept in the same bed, at age 4, and at age 11 he was fucking the family servants daily. He started visiting brothels at age 15 and daily at age 17. When he found out his mother was sleeping with one of his tutors he threatened to reveal all to his father if she didn't allow him to fuck her. She refused, he did as he threatened to do, and she killed herself [he was 13].

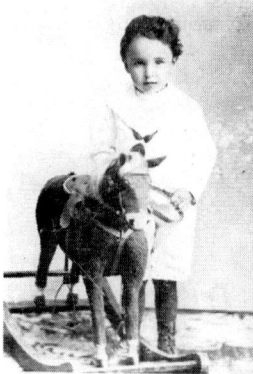

At age 3, a year before....

Reich fought in W.W. I and at age 22, while studying medicine, he met Freud who was so impressed by him that he gave Reich patients to analyze. Reich was accused of making his first patient pregnant and then of killing her in a botched abortion attempt. The girl's mother protested to the authorities and Reich claimed she did so because he had refused her sexual advances. She too committed suicide. Reich's biographer, Myron Sharaf, claimed Reich ordered other women and even his wives to have abortions, perhaps to spare him the cost of raising the children.

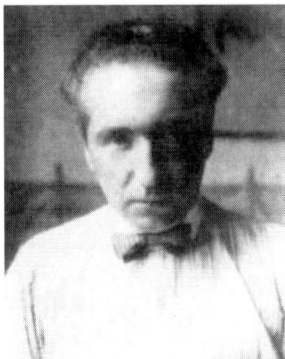

Reich around age 25.

He became a medical doctor and then studied neuropsychiatry under Nobel Prize Winner in Medicine Julius Wagner von Jauregg. He became an assistant director of Freud's Vienna clinic in 1924 at age 27. He gave seminars and his eloquence was described as enchanting and spellbinding. His presence and domination over others was, he himself wrote, ''like a shark in a pond of carps.''

He wrote erudite books extremely well received, especially by his mentor Freud, Freud who, incredibly, maintained that only men, not women, practiced autoerotism, and that the whole thing [masturbation] was ''infantile''.

He championed ''orgasmic potency'', stating that psychic health depended on the full discharge of the libido, that was ''not just fucking but included all of the excitation leading up to fucking'' [his words]. ''The more intense the preliminaries, the more intense is the orgasm, and the more satisfying and fulfilling the release.'' In this he was criticized, labeled the ''prophet of a better organism'', the ''founder of genital utopia'' and the man who believed that an orgasm was the solution to every neurosis.

He opened a number of clinics that gave free medical advice in contraception as well as psychoanalytic counseling, and he joined the Communist Party. His clinic became mobile. He drove into the suburbs and parks with a team of psychoanalysts and doctors, with advice, counsel and contraceptives. Even children were included in his effort at enlightenment, and teenagers encouraged to fully explore their sexuality. His promotion of teenage sex eventually got him excluded by the Danish Communist Party [Denmark, today, considered the world's happiest country, perhaps because it has (knowingly or not knowingly) incorporated certain of Reich's liberating concepts].

Reich had experiments using students in which they kissed and touched while Reich measured their body reactions on an oscillograph. One such student was the future chancellor Willy Brandt. Reich and his son spent a great deal of time looking for UFOs, and in America he invented the orgone accumulator in which the buyer--for example Norman Mahler [who owned several], Ginsberg, J.D. Salinger, Jack Kerouac and many others-- sat naked and were cured of cancer.

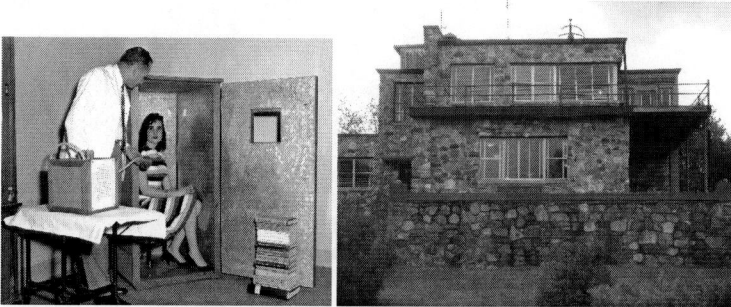

His Orgone Accumulator. His museum in Orgonon Maine

Imprisoned for being a charlatan, Reich was found dead in his cell, apparently of a heart attack.

1930 – F.W.W. Griffin, editor of *The Scouter*, wrote in a book aimed at Rover Scouts [a scout organization dedicated to older boys who had left the Boy Scouts, aged around 18-25] that masturbation was a ''natural stage of development.''

1970 – Thomas Szasz, psychiatrist and psychoanalyst stated that ''Masturbation is the primary sexual activity of mankind. In the nineteenth century it was a disease; in the twentieth, it's a cure.''

1972 – *Portnoy's Complaint* was banned in Australia because of things like this in Philip Roth's novel: ''That afternoon I came home from school to find my mother out of the house, and our refrigerator stocked with a big purplish piece of raw liver. I believe that I have already confessed to the piece of liver that I bought in a butcher shop and banged behind a billboard on the way to a bar mitzvah lesson. Well, I wish to make a clean breast of it. That wasn't my first piece. My first piece I had in the privacy of my own home, rolled around my cock in the bathroom at three-thirty, and then had again on the end of a fork, at five-thirty, along with the other members of that poor innocent family of mine. So. Now you know the worst thing I have ever done. I fucked my own family's dinner.''

1975 - Writer Michel Tournier wrote *The Meteors*: ''The brain provides the sexual organ with an imaginary object. This object rests with the hand to embody it. The hand is the ideal partner. Like an actor the hand plays the role it is given, but its masterpiece is masturbation. There it becomes at will either a penis or a vagina.''

1979 – A hardcore punk band called the Bedwetters came out with a first album they called Group Sex. In 1979 the name of the group was changed to Circle Jerks by vocalist Keith Morris.

1989 - Guillaume Fabert wrote in *Self-portrait of an Erection*, masturbation ''is to sex what aspirin is to medicine: *panacea*.''

1994 – The Surgeon General of the United States, Dr. Joycelyn Elders, was fired by President Clinton for suggesting that masturbation should be added to school curricula, and described as safe and healthy, as well as a means of having safe sex.

2006 – British Channel 4 sponsored Wank Week, with films and discussions, the program canceled due to protests.

2008 – A study at Tabriz Medical University found that ejaculations reduced swollen nasal blood vessels, freeing the airway for normal breathing, going so far as to suggest that ''the patient can adjust the number of intercourses or masturbations depending on the severity of the symptoms.''

2009 – The National Health Service in Sheffield England circulated a leaflet to parents, teachers and students stating that school children had a ''right'' to ''an orgasm a day'', adding that regular sex could be good for their cardiovascular health.

2009 – The Extremadura socialist government in Spain launched a €14,000 [$16,000] campaign aimed at children 14-17, its slogan: ''Pleasure is in your own hands.'' Leaflets, flyers and workshops instructed the young on self-pleasuring techniques, contraception and other forms of safe sex, over the objections of church officials and what they called ''conservative'' parents. The Barcelona *La Vanguardia* newspaper wrote that the Extremadura ''may have the most unemployed young people in Spain, but they will be the best at masturbation.''

2010 – The Supreme Court of Alabama upheld a state law criminalizing the distribution of sex-toys.

2013 – A Swede who openly masturbated on a beach in Sweden was cleared of charges of sexual assault, as the activity was not directed at another person.

2013 – Matthew Burdette, a San Diego High School student, committed suicide when a video of him masturbating in the school john went viral on the Net. ''I have no friends,'' he wrote in his suicide note. ''I don't want to kill myself but I have no friends.'' Matthew was 14.

2017 – A study by Harvard University indicated that men who masturbate 21 times a month or more have a 33% chance of NOT contracting prostate cancer.

CHAPTER ELEVEN

THE WORLD'S FOREMOST MASTURBATORS

Prince of Condé
1621-1686

Louis de Bourbon, Prince of Condé, was also known as the Duc d'Enghien and thanks to his military prowess, le Grand Condé. His father saw to his excellent education and at age 17 felt confident enough in the boy's abilities to turn over the governance of Burgundy to him, while he went off to war. Alas, his father also forced him to marry a woman all found homely and dull, simply because the girl was vaguely related to the all-important Cardinal Richelieu. The marriage nonetheless produced three children.

Condé's victories throughout Europe were stunning, and with the death of his father he became one of the wealthiest men in France, and earned the immensely prestigious title of *premier prince du sang*, which placed him in line for the throne itself, just after the son and grandson of the king.

Condé, through an extremely long career, found himself in a near limitless number of battles, at one time fighting to save Paris, at another he fought to capture the city, at one time he fought against the Spanish, at another with the Spanish against his own French. He was even imprisoned by the regent, Louis XIV's mother, and saved by the homely wife he had disgraced in words and body. His wounds were legend and in the Battle of Seneffe, against the Prince of Orange [later William III of England], he had three horses shot from under him.

He spent the last eleven years of his life in retirement in his Château de Chantilly, weakened from years of battle and sexual excess. He was omnisexual with a deep inclination for men and boys. Tallemant de Réaux, writer, memoirist and poet, was with Condé when he entered a tavern and, seeing ''*un jeune garcon qu'il trouvait charmant, l'entraine dans sa chambre*'' [''a charming youth, took him to his room.'']. Condé was dubbed the Great Masturbator because he loved to put his hand down men's trousers and bring them off while in conversation with them.

"Condé est un grand masterbateur qui met la main dans les chausses de tout homme qui lui plait." His favorites were his young pages, followed by his officers.

Another scene brought to us by Tallemant had Condé stopping at an inn where he met a charming schoolboy. He invited the lad to dinner and then to his room, a room that his lackeys immediately left because they knew what would be happening next. Condé asked the boy if he and his school friends jerked off, and without waiting for a response he plunge his hand down the boy's pants and said, surprised, "What! You don't have a hard-on?" *"Il plonge sa main dans la culotte du chérubin. Comment? Vous ne bandez pas!"* Condé then took out his dick and taught the boy how to jerk it with his left hand while plunging his right into Condé's ass *"et enseigne au novice à le branler de la main gauche en lui mettant les droits de la main droit dans le cul."*

He died of rheumatism and, it was said, a life of sexual pleasure.

Captain Robert Jones
1772

Because a man's life was at stake in Britain, sodomy had to be proved beyond doubt, making two concordant conditions imperative: The anus had to be proved to have been penetrated and sperm deposited therein, a seemingly impossible task until one reads the transcript of the trial of Robert Jones, in which one admires the prosecutor's thorough attempts to arrive at the truth, his in-depth questioning, and his success in bringing facts to light. The handling of the boy witness was exemplary, for the avuncular nature of the questioner visibly put the lad at ease, enough to detail acts made sordid due to the lad's extreme youth.

The boy had been 12 at the time, but because he was but a month from his 13th birthday, it is that age which is most often referred to. Had the acts taken place but a year later the consequences would have been greatly different, as the boy would have been 14, the age of consent in England [the act of *sodomy* remaining, nonetheless, punishable by hanging]. Because a man's life was in play, the interrogation had to be extremely precise and the boy's character beyond reproach. And indeed, the boy rose well above his contemporaries in that he was deemed by all who knew him as serious, trustworthy, scrupulously honest in speech, acts and testimony--and such was the lad's impact on the jury.

Puberty came later at that time than today, and the boy seemed to have been sexually indifferent to what he went through, himself incapable of being aroused or achieving orgasm. Had there been masturbation alone, Jones would have faced a simple misdemeanor.

The bare facts of the matter are these: The boy's uncle had a shop that did, among other things, shoe repairs. Captain Jones was a valued customer and had had ample opportunity to observe the lad. During one visit he suggested that the boy come to his residence in search of a pair of shoes in need of a new buckle. Because Jones's manner--open, warm and amusing--was appreciated by all, and because he was important to his uncle's affair, the boy was happy to consent--especially as there was the possibility that he could earn a coin or two.

Immediately on entering Jones's apartments Jones locked the door and proceeded to fondle the boy through his trousers, before lowering the boys pants and his own, preparatory to penetration, after which he apparently had a second orgasm by masturbating on the floor. The boy was requested to return the next morning where the man masturbated himself while fondling the boy, the whole scandal ending in a third visit where the same masturbatory act was repeated. The boy was paid all three times, trifling amounts in today's terms but back then a house could be rented for a shilling.

At home the lad fell ill and was bedded with pain between his thighs. Humiliated for what he had done for a few coppers, he kept the provenance of his suffering--the exact area and what had taken place--to himself.

Jones returned to the shop and requested that the boy deliver a pair of shoes he had ordered. When he left, the boy admitted to a friend of his uncle's that he didn't wish to go. The friend pursued the matter when the boy's uncle had left the shop on an errand, and the boy, yearning to get it off his chest, admitted all, the genesis of the trial and the following transcript. The boy's name is Hay:

Q. How old are you?

Hay. I shall be thirteen next January.

Q. Are you to tell the truth?

Hay. Yes.

Q. What do you know against the prisoner?

Hay. I live with my uncle a jeweler in Parliament Street. I met Captain Jones the prisoner, in St. Martin's Lane. He told me he had a buckle to mend.

Q. How long is that ago?

Hay. I believe about a month ago. He took me up stairs into his lodgings, in St. Martin's Court. He took me into his dining room, and he locked the door.

Q. Had you ever been in company with him before?

Hay. No. He always used to look at me, and give me halfpence when he met me. This time he pulled down my breeches and then his own.

Q. Were not you frightened at this?

Hay. Yes, I was a little. He set me in an elbow chair; he set me down and kissed me a little; then he made me lay down with my face on the chair, and so he came behind me; he put his cock into my hole.

Q. Did you submit to it quietly, or make any resistance?

Hay. I submitted to it quietly.

Q. How long might he keep it in your hole?

Hay. About five minutes I believe.

Q. Was he quite in?

Hay. A little.

Q. Was he in at all?

Hay. Yes.

Q. Did you find anything come from him?

Hay. Some wet stuff that was white; I wiped it off.

Q. Can you describe to the jury how far it was in your body?

Hay. No.

Q. What did you wipe the wet off with?

Hay. My shirt.

Q. You are sure it was in you?

Hay. Yes.

Q. What did he do after this?

Hay. He spouted some on the ground.

Q. Did he spout some into your hole?

Hay. Yes.

Q. What did he do after this?

Hay. He set me down in the elbow chair, kissed me a little, and gave me some halfpence and told me not to tell anybody.

Q. How long did you stay?

Hay. About half an hour.

Q. Did he attempt to do anything more to you?

Hay. No, not then.

Q. How came you not to cry out?

Hay. I was ashamed.

Q. Had ever anybody served you in this manner before?

Hay. No.

Q. Did you tell your uncle, or anybody, when you came home?

Hay. No.

Q. How soon did you go again?

Hay. He desired me to come next day; I went; he unbuttoned my breeches again, and then his own.

Q. What time did you go next day?

Hay. About eleven o'clock. He made me rub his cock up and down till some white stuff came again.

Q. At the time he put his cock into your hole, it was stiff and hard, was it?

Hay. Yes.

Q. Did he attempt anything behind then?

Hay. No.

Q. How long did you stay with him then?

Hay. About ten minutes.

Q. You quietly submitted to all that?

Hay. Yes. He gave me the buckle and some halfpence then, and desired me to come again next day; I went next day about eleven o'clock. He unbuttoned his breeches again, and mine too. He did the same again that time as he did the last day.

Q. What happened next?

Hay. I was taken very ill after this. I was ill a week. I had a pain in my thighs and legs that I could not stand. About a fortnight ago, after I was well, he came to the shop one day, and looked on the show glasses. He bespoke a shirt buckle of my uncle. It was to be sent home to him. My uncle ordered me to go with the buckle. I told him he had better go, and perhaps he might get the captain's business.

Q. When you went so willingly two days together after the first offence was committed, how came you to make the objection to go now?

Hay. I was afraid he would serve me the same thing again.

Q. How came you to object to go now and not before?

Hay. He told me not to tell of it, and I was ashamed. The reason was because I was so ill.

Q. Did you think you had been doing a wrong thing?

Hay. Yes. As soon as he left the shop I told Mr. Rapley of it. He is a jeweler.

Q. What time was it the captain came to look at the show glass?

Hay. About twelve o'clock.

Q. How came you to tell Mr. Rapley, and not tell your uncle?

Hay. I was ashamed to tell my uncle.

Q. Did you go there before dinner?

Hay. Yes.

Q. Did you tell your uncle the whole story, how he had served you these three times?

Hay. I told him what he had done to me the first time, but not the last times.

Q. How came you to tell it now, when you kept it a secret so long.

Hay. I thought I would tell of it all the while, but I was ashamed.

Q. Did you think you had been doing a wrong thing with him.

Hay. Yes.

Q. Then how came you to go of your own accord the second and third times?

Hay. I thought my uncle might get business by it.

Q. Did anything more happen than what you have told us now?
Hay. No.

The newspapers related that it took the jury 5 minutes to reach a decision, death by hanging, a verdict later rescinded in exchange for Jones's exile from England, for which he was allowed two weeks. The clemency granted by the king was due to a petition by a large number of notables who vouched for Jones's character, with the exception of this brief error in judgment. In reality, Jones--like a huge percentage of the English who had undergone boyhood boarding-school adventures--was bisexual, and it was most probable that usually Jones found contentment with adolescents, not prepubescent children like Hay.

One paper claimed he went to Florence for a time, not the worst of exiles, and then to Lyons where, said another paper, he lived with his footboy [male domestic worker]. He was reported as going to Turkey where he served assorted Beys, but during a conflict that arose between several pretenders to the throne, he championed the wrong side and had his head separated from his body.

[For much more, see my book *British Homosexuality*.]

Marquis de Sade
1740-1814

The story of the life of de Sade begins in 1940 when his surviving papers were discovered by a relative, Comte Xavier de Sade, who came across the documents of an ancestor he'd never heard of, a name passed over in silence for nearly 150 years, erased from the collective memory. The documents Xavier de Sade found were the remnants of de Sade's literary output, most destroyed at his death by his son, the rest lost in the 18th and 19th centuries.

The words sadism and sadist come from de Sade's name, sadistic crimes for which he would be put in prison or in asylums for 32 years of his life. The first major scandal came when he was 28, reported by a woman who had escaped from the de Sade chateau after being tortured and whipped. The *Revue de Paris* published an article in 1837 that claimed that de Sade, armed with chocolates and Spanish Fly, went to Marseille where he used the Spanish-Fly-drugged chocolates in a brothel, as well as wine, the result an orgy the *Revue* called as great as ''the bacchantes of antiquity'', during which two girls died in the frenzy, one of whom ''hurled herself out of a window'', while ''the Marquis de Sade and his valet ran off.'' He and his manservant were sentenced to death for the poisoning and for sodomy [which they practiced together and on others], but both fled to Italy.

De Sade returned to his chateau where his physical and sexual abuses against his employees was such that one father came to free his daughter and attempted to shoot de Sade in the face, but the gun misfired. He was finally captured under his death warrant and sent to the Bastille where he began *The 120 Days of Sodom* and other works, until the storming of the Bastille during the French Revolution of 1789. Freed, he began publishing his works anonymously and in 1801 Napoleon ordered his arrest for publishing filth. In jail his ardor at seducing young prisoners was such that he was judged insane and put away in an asylum.

De Sade had been raised by an uncle after his father abandoned the family and his mother entered a convent. He was indulged by his servants who met his every whim, which encouraged his rebelliousness and unrestrained temper. He went to the Lycée Louis-le-Grand in Paris, one of the very best, where his uncontrolled temper and rampant sexuality were met by sever corporal punishment, involving whippings, and this before age 14. He entered a military academy and was commissioned a sub-lieutenant at age 15. He became a colonel and fought in the Seven Years' War. He married and had two sons and a daughter.

He died at age 74 in the Charenton Lunatic Asylum in 1814. His request to be buried without religious ceremony was denied.

Oscar Wilde
1854-1909

Oscar Wilde took a huge part of his pleasure in masturbating, his preferred form of sex, often consisting of two boys on a bed making love, while he observed, jerking off.

No boy had had a more auspicious beginning that Oscar Wilde. Born rich, surrounded by servants, a German governess and French maid, physically he was not one of the boys that other boys--deadly serious about their sex--fought over in the boarding schools Wilde was packed off to (16), boys they possessed at night until the next pretty face came along. Wilde's personality became flippant, as a way of compensating for his lack of looks, his big, awkward body too padded to be erotically attractive, too ungainly, a face too homely. He therefore overcompensated, as do actors: jackets with large checkers, bright ties, high collars, huge hats rakishly tilted over one or the other ear.

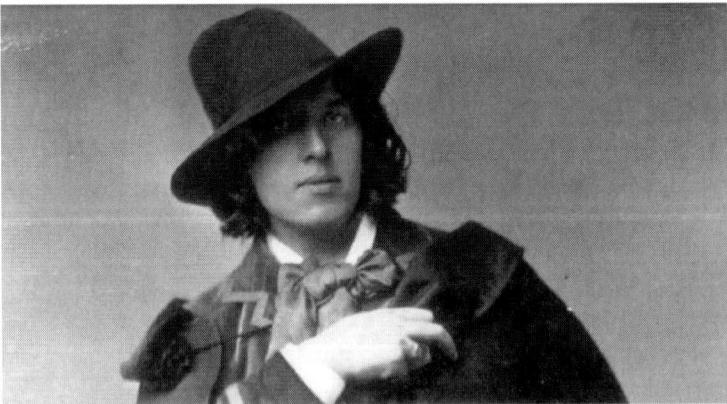
Everything about Wilde was exaggerated.

Wilde at first toyed with heterosexuality. A marriage produced two sons, Cyril and Vyvyan, whose last names were changed to Holland after Wilde's trial for sodomy. Both were educated in Switzerland. Cyril became an army captain and served in India before being killed by a sniper in W.W. I. His son Vyvyan served in both World Wars and died at age 80. Both sons were prevented by law from ever seeing their father again, although Vyvyan accompanied his father's remains to his last resting place, at the side of Wilde's last lovers, Douglas and Robert Ross.

In 1886 Wilde had met 17-year-old Robert Ross who, enamored of his poetry, seduced his hero, Wilde, age 32. Robbie Ross, age 24 in this picture, remained Wilde's loyal friend until Wilde's death, aiding him financially. He became Wilde's legal executor and made sure that Wilde's two boys received the royalties from his books. Openly gay, Ross was a journalist and art critic. He had had sexual relations with a boy of 16 who admitted to sleeping with Lord Alfred Douglas in Ross's home, but the boy's parents, to avoid scandal, did not press charges. He died in 1918. In 2008 the University of Bradford named its library collection the Robbie Ross Liberation Library.

In 1889 he met John Gray, 23, the lad who became his *Dorian Gray*. At the time it was extraordinary for a poor boy to work himself into the upper-classes, something Gray did, starting out as a carpenter at age 18, learning French, German and Latin on his own, succeeding in Civil Service examinations which opened the ranks of government employment, and then his meeting with Wilde and their sexual union. *The Portrait of Dorian Gray* came out in 1890. In the book Gray goes on to ever-mounting perversion, as did Wilde, and, later, from prison Wilde wrote Douglas that he should have been wise enough to remain with Gray or someone like him. Amusingly, W.H. Smith refused to sell *The Portrait of Dorian Gray*, calling it filth.

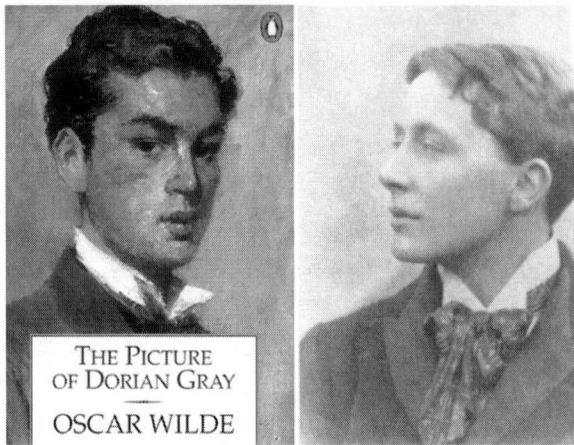
Dorian Gray book jacket and John Gray.

He came across what he considered the faultless beauty of Douglas in 1890, a budding poet at Oxford, whom Wilde was said to have worshipped. Both liked teenage male prostitutes, and both had the means to assuage their desires. Their degeneracy was total, but degeneracy is what very man wishes for himself sometime in his life. Both Douglas and Wilde played Douglas's mother and father for fools because neither guessed what was going on, as parents do not generally raise their boys to be sodomised, especially not by flabby, faded lechers like Wilde.

In 1895 Douglas's father the Marquess of Queensbury left a card at Wilde's residence addressed ''To Oscar Wilde, ponce and somdomite,'' misspelling the word in his fury. Wilde had the Marquess arrested and charged with criminal libel. Frank Harris, the famous author of the highly pornographic *My Life and Loves*, and Bernard Shaw, told him that if he didn't drop the proceedings he would be destroyed. Wilde, the now most famous playwright in England, was too disdainful to heed the supplications. He would pay with his life, for from then onwards an early death was the direction his destiny took.

During his trial the Marquess said he lived for one reason, to save his son. And it may have been the truth. The boys called on to testify to Wilde being a sodomite were so numerous that when the Marquess was pronounced innocent the court irrupted in applause. Wilde himself was immediately incarcerated. Wilde's trial brought more witnesses against him, one who maintained ''He told me to come into his bedroom and worked me up with his hand and made me spend in his mouth.'' Hotel staff commented on the boys in his bed, the fecal stains and vaseline-stiff sheets, resulting in Wilde being sentenced to two years of hard labor.

Once released from jail Wilde returned to Douglas, in Capri (20), and then on to Paris, the greatest city in the world when one is young, as I well know having spent a third of my life there. But Wilde was penniless and haggard. It was then he said, ''The cruelty of a prison sentence starts when you come out.''

The Marquess of Queensbury died in 1900, requesting to be cremated and that ''no Christian tomfooleries'' were to be performed, my own wish exactly. He left £20,000 to his son Douglas, a part of which Wilde asked Douglas to turn over to him, stating that he deserved it. Douglas disagreed. Wilde died in the same year as the Marquess. He maintained that he had lived and died for love, which, in our imperfect world, could conceivably mean fecal-stained and vaseline-stiff sheets.

[The full story of Wilde's life can be found in my book *The History of British Homosexuality*.]

Proust
1871-1922

Marcel Proust [Valentin Louis Georges Eugène Marcel Proust, 1871-1922] was raised in the Catholic faith of his father, a pathologist and epidemiologist, while his mother, issued from a wealthy Jewish family, instilled the love of literature in Proust. He went to the Lycée Condorcet, along with some of France's foremost writers like Cocteau and Verlaine, and other students who introduced him into the spheres of the upper bourgeoisie, the subject of his *magnum opus, À la recherche du temps perdu.* He finished his education at the Sorbonne with a degree in law in 1893 and in philosophy in 1895.

Few people had as tangled a character as did Proust. Ultra-conservative, a snob for whom only the wealthy classes existed [so unlike Zola who frequented all stratums, and whose *Bête humaine* and *Au Bonheur des Dames* are as pleasurable to read today as when they were first written]. Proust was by nature an enemy of socialism and believed that there should be no division between church and state, as the church offered structure and stability, yet he was personally an atheist. Physically in poor health, he nonetheless completed his military service, which he later called paradise thanks to the working-class boys he met there. Afterwards, when his father insisted that he do something worthwhile with his life, he worked as a volunteer in the Bibliotèque Mazarine, living at home until the death of both his parents, who left him financially independent. Paradoxically, he was considered lazy in the execution of his art, while leaving us with an immense *oeuvre*, writing that took place at night during his last years, coming to an end when he died of pneumonia.

His greatest literary influence was Scotsman John Ruskin, 1819-1900, the da Vinci of the 1800s, whose mind encompassed art, geology, myth, literature, botany, economy and even fairy tales to name but a few of his interests, which he put in books and conferences. His influence on Proust and Proust's contemporaries was incalculable, and Proust, aided by his mother [who was bilingual], translated a number of his works into French. Proust was also influenced by Saint-Simon, Montaigne, Stendhal, Flaubert, Dostoyevsky and Tolstoy. He started *À la recherche du temps perdu* at age 38 and died at age 51, the last 3 volumes of the total of 7 were proofread and published posthumously by his brother Robert, in all approximately 3,200 pages in French, 4,300 in the English translation. Homosexuality is discussed in his book, but Proust never admitted to being homosexual, just as most men at the time hid theirs too, Montherlant, Jouhandeau and Gide [until the end of Gide's life], while Cocteau had the honesty and courage of his sexuality. [Gide's book *Corydon* was nonetheless published *after* Proust's *Sodom and Gomorra* which, claimed Gide, gave him the mettle to release his book.]

Until the advent of liberating Internet, masturbation haunted the lives of sons and fathers, some to the point of despair. At age 16 Proust's father gave him 10 francs as payment for a prostitute who would make a man of him and break his excessive masturbation. Proust was unable to go through with it the first time so he asked his grandfather for 10 more francs in order to give it a second try, as ''it cannot happen twice in a lifetime that a person is too flustered to screw'', he wrote in an extremely open letter.

We don't know with how many male students Proust had sex, but he did write letters to his good friend Daniel Halévy, later a writer and biographer, and Jacques Bizet, son of the famous composer who died when Jacques was only 3, letters explicitly asking for sex and stating that if the boys didn't help relieve him his only recourse was masturbation, adding that he'd been caught by his father, the explanation for the above 10 francs. At the time [and right up to my generation] masturbation was considered harmful for both the body and a boy's morals, and led directly to homosexuality. Both Halévy and Bizet declined to give Proust a hand, probably because of a lack of sexual attraction to Proust, as well as Proust's arrogance and his need to ever dominate those with whom he came into contact. His classmates were convinced he was spoiled, while Proust maintained he was trapped in a form of parental slavery. Proust certainly participated in circle jerks at school urinals, and Montherlant wrote that he'd been beaten up when he refused such activity. [In French schools the urinals were/are outside, in the playgrounds, modestly protected from view by a sheet of metal that rises from the knees to the lower shoulders, making both pissing and mutual masturbation undetectable if the boys look straight ahead, viewing the others by moving only the eyes. The action was/is mostly solo.]

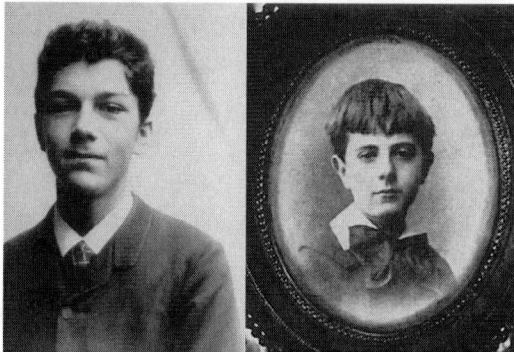

Daniel Halévy and Jacques Bizet around the ages when

Proust desired them.

In 1895 Proust, age 22, dedicated a short story to a boy of 19, Reynaldo Hahn, a musician with whom he traveled and took the female role of Swann's love Odette in Proust's book.

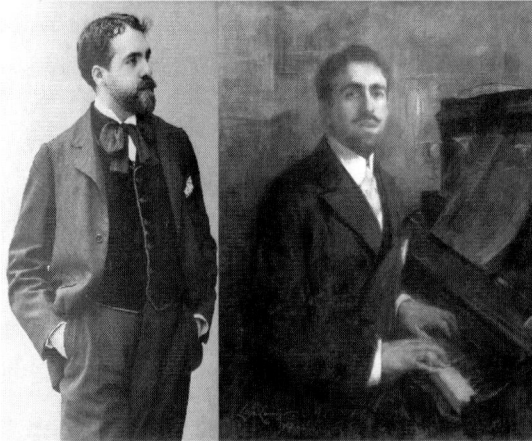

Reynaldo Hahn, the painting by Lucie Lambert.

At the end of 1895 Proust met the effeminate, androgynous Lucien Daudet, age 16, and both hit it off to the extent that they were seen merrily giggling together, mutual happiness that led to tense relations between Proust and Montesquiou. Now, Montesquiou was as sissyish as Proust and Lucien, a man who loved to give soirées which were luxurious and beautifully catered to, and the people invited were the *crème-de-la-crème*. Both Proust and Lucien were summoned to one and Proust, in his letter of acceptance, told Montesquiou that he and Lucien couldn't be in each other's company without breaking up in laughter, and that Lucien's father, the eminent writer Alphonse Daudet, with whom both were staying, had had to put up with them, and warned Montesquiou that he would have to do so too. Montesquiou was furious because he had the premonition that this was a conspiracy of Proust's to ruin Montesquiou's dinner, simply because Proust was jealous of Montesquiou's successful and often publicized gatherings. When both boys did arrive, Montesquiou's severity had them ''bent over into peals of laughter, and they had to rush out of the room, gasping for air. Montesquiou *never* forgave them for this impropriety," a story brought to us by William C. Carter in his wonderful *Proust in Love*, 2006.

The incredible hubbub of the Proust-Lucien Daudet relationship found its way into the papers when writer Jean Lorrain penned an acid chronicle revealing their "friendship". Although Lorrain was as effeminate as Proust and Lucien [and Montesquiou], he thought himself sexually superior because instead of the poufs the others went with, Lorrain specialized in more masculine types, sailors and male hustlers [which at times led to his being beaten up]. The article, in *Le Journal,* began by stating that Proust's just-published *Les plaisirs et les jours* was written by a sissy for sissies, and that Proust's next book of poems would be prefaced by the renowned Alphonse Daudet because he could never refuse a request of his son, Lucien, which meant, to those attuned to such things, that Proust was sleeping with the young and handsome Lucien.

Lorrain and Proust faced off in a duel in the woods of Medon, in the early morning. Legend has it that one of Proust's lovers, a hairdresser, rushed forward and threw himself at Proust's feet, begging him to not go through with it. By common agreement both Lorrain and Proust had pledged to shoot into the ground, and as no one outside of Proust, Lorrain and their seconds knew about the agreement, every major newspaper article concerning both underlined their courage. The men left the field without shaking hands only because their seconds discouraged an overt display of connivance, and for the rest of Proust's life he took the opportunity, during every dinner he was invited to, to vaunt his fearless behavior.

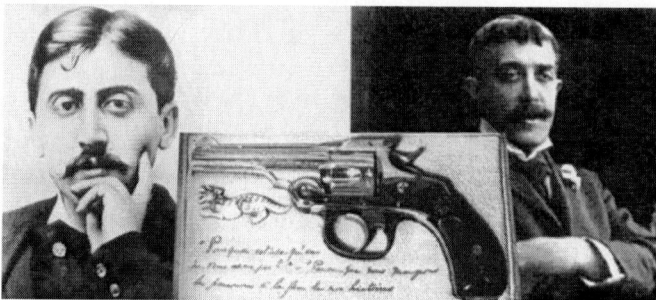

Proust/Lorrain duel.

It was the discovery of the real beauty of boys during Proust's military service, so unlike the perfumed and jeweled dandies he had largely known until then, that made him prefer servants and working-class lads, whorehouse hustlers, sailors and soldiers, always for pay, to the point that he would himself advance the funds for the establishment of at least two male brothels.

In 1908 the Eulenburg scandal irrupted, involving Kaiser Wilhelm II and several Prussians (13), and of course there had been the Oscar Wilde trial and disgrace (7), which posed no threat to Proust as homosexuality had not been punished in France since 1791, after the Revolution. Besides hustlers and visits to male brothels, Proust hired men to provide him with boys, men who were servants in cafés, cabarets and even the Ritz, and many of the boys may have been underage, under 21 at that time. [Male homosexual acts were illegal until 1791. The age of consent was set at age 11 in 1832, at 13 in 1863 and 21 for homosexual act during Proust's lifetime. It was lowered to 18 in 1974 and has been age 15 since 1982.] Proust therefore thought he could be imprisoned, whereas in reality men like Proust, Gide and Montherlant, as well as many actors, were fully known to the police who went out of their way to turn a blind eye. Paris was a homosexual paradise during the Belle Époque (18), especially for the well-off and for tourists, notably Brits and Americans. Gide, Montherlant and Proust had nothing to worry about, but they didn't know it. Of course, their belief that they could be arrested for having sex with underage lads added piquancy to their liaisons, needed spice when otherwise they could have as many encounters as they could pay for.

Gide dismissed Proust's work as fictionalized gossip, which was true of Truman Capote too, who is not only America's greatest homosexual writer, but, for some like me, the greatest American writer to have lived. This could have been Proust's destiny also had he come clean about his life, as Capote had his own, instead of disguising his homosexual male characters. Allusions to homosexual acts are as difficult to find as diamonds in Proust's book, as when Mme Verdun put two musicians in communicating bedrooms and told them, "If you want to have a little music don't worry about us, the walls are as thick as a fortress," apparently giving them permission to fuck their brains out.

Proust had two major sources of information for his books and for sex. One was the Ritz Hotel where the *maître d'hôtel*, Olivier Dabescot, and the hotel personnel, lavishly paid by Proust, met in a room put at Proust's disposal where they filled the writer in on the hotel guests and their sexual proclivities. As the waiters were chosen for their beauty, their knowledge came from often-intimate contact with the hotel guests, and those Proust personally favored could be invited to dine with him and spend time on the accompanying couch, the obligatory fixture in the private dining rooms.

The second source of information came from Albert Le Cuziat who owned several male brothels with baths, the most noted of which was the Ballon d'Alsace, frequented by deputies, ministers, officers and the upper bourgeoisie.

French writer Marcel Jouhandeau recounted exactly how Proust found pleasure in male brothels, brought to us by William Carter: On entering the establishment Proust would go to a door through which he could see but not be seen by the group of boys inside playing cards. Proust would choose one and then go to an upstairs room and slip naked in bed, drawing the sheet up to his chin. The boy chosen would go into the room and, following the brothel owner's instructions, strip naked and jerk himself to orgasm, while Proust did the same under the sheet. As soon as the boy came he was told to smile and then leave. If Proust had reached orgasm he would dress and also leave, if not an extremely unfortunate scene took place: the brothel owner would enter with two famished rats in separate cages. He would put the cages together and open the doors. The rats would attack each other, squealing and spewing blood, which caused Proust to ejaculate. By this time, old and ill, Proust had a Howard-Hughes phobia of germs that excluded any physical contact with another [as his father had been an epidemiologist, Proust had learned, young, to fear germs].

William Carter ends his book on Proust in a way that may inspire the reader to give Proust's Everest a try, or a second chance if he hadn't been able to get as far as the base camp during a previous reading: "*In Search of Lost Time* is, to my mind, comedy of the highest order that amuses, delights, and frequently dazzles as we follow the Narrator on his quest. After many ups and downs and wrong turns, the story has a happy ending in which the myriad themes--major and minor--beautifully orchestrated throughout, are gloriously resolved in the grand finale." (21)

Jacques d'Adelswärd-Fersen
1880 - 1923

During the time of Jacques d'Adelswärd-Fersen [whom I'll call Fersen from hereon], rich boys often turned to writing poetry to justify their existence, something Byron did. It is extremely difficult to judge their works because in modern times we need a Rosetta Stone to understand what they were trying to reveal to us, as illustrated by this poem by Shelley, supposed to be the best description of an orgasm ever written:

The Serchio, twisting forth
Between the marble barriers which it clove
At Ripafratta, leads through the dread chasm
The wave that died the death which lovers love,
Living in what it sought; as if this spasm
Had not yet passed, the toppling mountains cling,
But the clear stream in full enthusiasm
Pours itself on the plain.

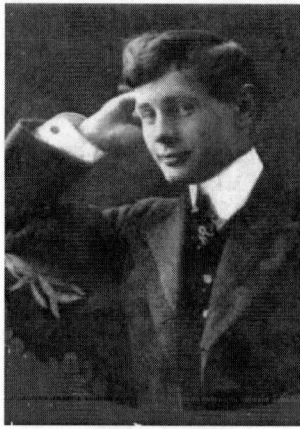

Fersen

Born in Paris in 1880, Fersen's grandfather, a Swedish count, founded a steel industry at Longwy in the east of France, which Fersen inherited at age 22, his father having died at age 40, perhaps of yellow fever contracted in Panama, when Fersen was seven. Fersen had a brother, Renold, who died young. Both father and brother were greatly loved by Fersen, if one can judge from the characters in his books, often named Axel after his father, and Renold. Fersen went to Science-Po in Paris, its best school then as today, and the University of Geneva. His literary reputation resides on his *oeuvre*, ten collections of poems, three novels and the creation of a literary review called *Akademos*.

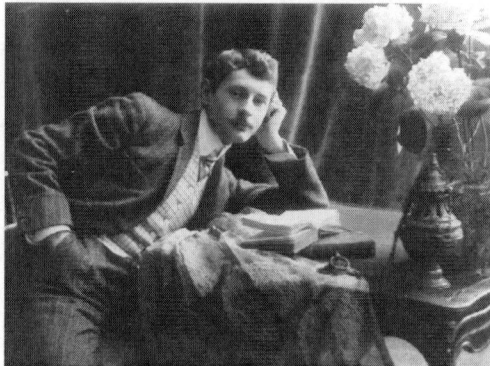

Fersen

His best friend and lover was Hans de Warren, a school chum with whom he would pick up boys, often directly as they left their *lycées*, at times in parks. The lads were invited home to Fersen's wealthy residence near the Arc de Triomphe after a joyride in the family royal-blue Darracq, driven by a liveried chauffeur. There the boys were offered cakes and wine, shown Fersen and Warren's extensive collection of pornography, and, thusly excited, they were masturbated and blown. There is no record of anal sex, but the subject would have been avoided by police investigators as grossly unpleasant, or referred to in such general terms as to make denial easy, to the relief of the offenders and the questioners. One of the boys confessed that Fersen drew a picture of his penis, and he measured that of another, hard. A third lad said that after inhaling ether and ingesting morphine, Fersen, misty-eyed, proposed that they both go to Venice where he would give the boy half his fortune, and where they would die in a suicide pact.

All of this came out after the incident that brought both Fersen and Warren to trial. Both boys, in their early twenties, organized living tableaux that they put on in front of an audience. The actors in the tableaux were all young boys, from age 7 to 17, the average being 14. The seven-year-old had an extremely early sexual awakening, thanks to his brothers who were participants, and whose talk and nightly masturbation filled him in on adolescent sex. During the tableaux the boys took poses while poetry was read. The boys, as well as the audience, were made up of the crème of Parisian society, the boys coming from the very best families and schools, the audience composed of men--but some women--estimated as 70% pederastic. During the tableaux one of the boys would always be naked, his privates covered by gauze if seen frontally, his buttock *au naturel* if lying on a couch or the floor. Afterwards they would retire to the bathroom to clean up. Aroused by their performance, they gratefully allowed the two older boys to masturbate and blow them. Fersen and Warren would also allow themselves to be manipulated until ejaculation.

The séances went on twice a week, Thursdays and Sundays, until the father of the seven-year-old found out and demanded that the police arrest Fersen and Warren, threatening, when they hesitated because of the families involved, to go public if they didn't. They did, but he went public anyway, and the resultant scandal was horrendous. The seven-year-old and his two brothers must have gone through hell at the hand of their daddy, but of this we know nothing.

Fersen was examined by three psychiatrists, one of which *purportedly* diagnosed him with inherited insanity, alcoholism and epilepsy. A physician, Doctor Socquet, found he had scabies [a contagious skin infection caused by mites] and gonorrhea, and the judge questioning him, as well as his clerk, were said to have gone to public baths after each interrogation to avoid contamination [private bathrooms in one's apartment were still rare at the time].

A fictional account of the tableaux, called Black Masses in the press, came out in 1904, written by the pornographer Alphonse Gallais, *Les Mémoires du Baron Jacques*, in which Baron Jacque's mother takes his virginity at an early age. Baron Jacques goes on to deflower his own young boys, copulating with them on his mother's skeleton!

For Fersen's times what he did was highly titillating, and because minors were involved he was sentenced to five months in prison. As he was no longer welcome by family and friends, he exchanged Paris's cloudy skies for sunny Capri. But before we get to his exploits there, perhaps a word on his *oeuvre*.

In 1902 he published a collection of poems called *L'Hymnaire d'Adonis*, in which we find the poem *Treize Ans*: At age 13, blond with precocious eyes full of desire and emotion, his lips already streetwise, he's in his school study hall where all the boys are reading, bent over their books, while only he, in a corner, is going through randy poems by Musset. As the supervisor goes by he hides what he's doing and pretends to be hard at work, but when the coast's clear he brings out his book and, turning into the shadows so as not to be seen, he slips his hand into his pocket where a hole leads to his toy that, lost in licentious thoughts, he fondles for a long, long time. [*Treize ans, blondin aux yeux précoces, Qui disent le désir et l'émoi, Lèvres, ayant je ne sais quoi De mutin, de vicieux, de gosse. Il lit; dans la salle ils sont Tous penchés à écrire un thème, Lui seul dans un coin lit quand même, Des vers de Musset, polissons; Le pion passe, vite il se cache, Semblant travailler avec feu, À quelque devoir nébuleux, Très propre, soigné et sans tache, Puis calmé, le moment d'après, Reprend tout rose sa lecture, Se met à changer de posture, Pour être de l'ombre plus près; Coule ses mains, sans qu'on devine, Dans sa poche percée d'un trou, Et là longuement fait joujou, Rêveur de voluptés félines!*]

Rich but rejected, Fersen withdrew to Capri, noted for being a homosexual refuge since Tiberius withdrew there 2000 years previously (20). Fersen built a palace, the Villa Lysis, facing Tiberius' Villa Jovis, a neoclassical affair of Ionic columns, an entrance with an atrium, and bedrooms with wondrous views of the palace gardens, the distant sea and Mount Vesuvius. There he surrounded himself with island boys until he was requested to leave when he brought in boys from elsewhere, in competition with the homegrown crop, a loss of income for the lads and their families. The Caprian boys in question have been immortalized by a succession of painters and photographers, the most noted of whom was Wilhelm von Gloeden, their bodies caressed by generations of financially fortunate lovers of boys (20).

A basement apartment, called the Chinese Room, was dedicated to opium smoking, where Fersen contented himself with up to 40 pipes a day, a huge but supposedly not unheard-of quantity for addicts. Opium depresses the urge to have sex, although it can be used to postpone an orgasm, allowing more enjoyment before eventual ejaculation. Taking 40 pipes meant he was having no orgasms at all. It was in the Chinese Room that, in 1923, at age 43, his health failing, he drank a mortal cocktail of cocaine and champagne, certainly entering eternity with an ecstatic Wow!

[For far more, see my book *French Homosexuality*.]

Duncan Grant
1885-1978

Duncan Grant was born in England but as a baby he was taken to India where, thanks to his father's rank in the army, he was surrounded by servants, servants that even bachelor soldiers could offer themselves, a sepoy to hand even a corporal his soap in the shower, another his towel, each careful not to infringe on the work of the other, as it was their only means of livelihood. The heat was debilitating, and only at the end of the afternoons did the soldiers leave their beds in preparation for the evening meal and drink that would plunge them into welcome oblivion. Military exercises were few and the favorite pastime was pig sticking. Relief could be found in the mountains, especially in Casmir (21).

At age 9 Duncan returned to England to begin his formal schooling. His mother's sister-in-law, Jane Strachey, Lady Strachey, had a hand in finding a school for him, Hillbrow, where she sent her own son James, two years younger than Duncan, a boy who would become one of Duncan's lovers, although James's older brother Lytton would have Duncan first. At Hillbrow Duncan was popular, largely due to his having lived in India and the tales of his sojourn there, and he was good at sports, always a way into the group that held the most power in prep schools. James Strachey was his best friend and he knew Rupert Brooke, also attending the school. The headmaster, Mr. Eden, liked to birch boys and fondle the younger ones in their baths, until a boy told his father and Eden was expulsed. Duncan recounted that Rupert went to the headmaster and helped him pack to leave, something Duncan was certain had saved Eden's life, as he had contemplated suicide until Rupert showed his compassion, Rupert only 15 at the time, already levelheaded--so much promise extinguished by his early death (7).

Douglas Blair Turnbaugh, in his excellent *Duncan Grant and the Bloomsbury Group*, 1987, relates a segment of Duncan's life that freed him from religious nonsense and got him thinking independently, all thanks to James Strachey. Duncan had been to a church service where he had the vision of Christ coming down the aisle and laying hands on him. He told James who suggested they look up Christianity in the *Encyclopedia Britannica*. We don't know which passage the boys read, but James asked, "Do you mean to say you believe all this?" Wrote Duncan later: "My Christianity fell away from me like a mantle." Nietzsche too had removed the shackles of superstition very young. Nietzsche wrote, "God, the immortality of the soul, redemption, the 'beyond' were concepts I had no time to pay attention to--not even as a child, perhaps because I wasn't childish enough. I was too curious, too questioning, too exuberant to put up with a concept as crude as the existence of a god. For me, God was an invitation *to not think*."

Duncan stayed with the Stracheys until his parents returned from Rangoon. It was at Hillbrow prep school that his talent for art was first recognized and encouraged, followed, at age 14, by St. Paul's day school. He took military training but was found inept, always dropping his rifle, and in his studies he was branded an imbecile, especially due to his complete ignorance in mathematics [which didn't stop him from having his affair with the mathematical genius, Keynes, and become the love of Keynes's life]. In fact, he was found only suited for art, notably after he won prizes that St. Paul's offered in painting. At age 17 he went to the Westminster School of Art, taking up residence with the Stracheys in a seven-storey home Duncan's mother Ethel called a palace. She and Duncan's father Bartle were housed there too on occasion, in a hugely numerous family, a building that was vast, albeit with only one bathroom.

A revealing incident took place when he was 17. He had been sent to the South of France where, on the way, in Paris, he bought a book *How We Lost Our Virginity*, exactly what a young lad would buy and of course use to stimulate masturbation, although not that much outward stimulation was necessary in pre-pornography years when a bare shoulder, or an ankle or bicep [depending on one's sexual bent] could spurn crazed episodes of self-abuse, as it was called at the time.

Lytton Strachey was five years older than Duncan, a student of Trinity College, Cambridge. Cambridge had freed his mind intellectually and unbridled his sexuality. Lady Strachey had spent a great deal of her life in India, her father in the government and her future husband, Richard, one of his secretaries, both serving during the horrific Mutiny of 1857 (21). Lady Strachey had lost an eye, and had trained herself in Braille as she knew she was losing sight in the other, something that tells us a great deal about the force of nature found in all the Stracheys. She was a feminist, and intellectually suited to accept her two sons' homosexuality.

Duncan went to day schools and so may have escaped early carnal knowledge, common in boarding schools (16). He later recalled his first sexual experience to the love of the last half of his life, Paul Roche. He was in the National Gallery looking at a painting when an older boy came up behind him, reached around and gently rubbed his penis through his trousers. ''We were alone in the room--he pulled out my cock and very soon I came onto the floor. I rubbed the mess with my foot.'' The boy was a Swede that Duncan greatly liked and rendezvoused with several times. When the Swede left, Duncan wondered if he could produce the same sensation on his own. He did to himself what the Swede had done and came, his first experience with masturbation. From then on the floodgates were open.

Duncan's book on how to lose one's virginity was discovered and the boy was sent to a series of doctors because the adults were certain he was on the edge of dementia, until finally he had the good fortune of finding a doctor who told him he had nothing to worry about, that, in other words, his playing with himself was of no consequence. The story is important because even without the doctor's council, Duncan was a boy who had, from an extremely early age, accepted himself, accepted his sexuality and shucked religious voodooism.

[Duncan Grant's full life can be found in my book *The Bloomsbury Set*.]

Maynard Keynes
1883-1946

At this very moment, somewhere in the world, economists and philosophers have the name of John Maynard Keynes on their lips, perhaps furiously in favor of his ideas, perhaps furiously against, but all are as respectful as before an ancient god. Among the Bloomsbury Setters, he is by far the shining light. He saw to the Sets creature comforts, and stepped in when the power of the government, legal advice, guarantees for loans, help in the purchase of homes and land, were required. He provided Duncan

Grant with an annuity, and most certainly aided others in need, backstage, out of love and humanism. We have every reason to get to know this truly exceptional human being.

It was Keynes who was the first to spearhead, in the 1930s, the then-revolutionary idea of free markets. Keynes fought for virile intervention in fiscal and monetary policies, thanks to which the disaster of 1929 came to an end, as well as the world financial crises of 2007-2008.

In 1990 TIME magazine wrote, ''his radical idea that governments should spend money they don't have may have saved capitalism.''

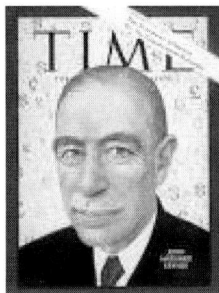

Keynes made the cover of TIME on the 31st of December 1965. TIME wrote, ''We are all Keynesians now.''

Keynes was born in Cambridge, Cambridgeshire, to upper-middle-class parents, his father an economist and lecturer at Cambridge, his mother a social reformer, the perfect storm in the creation of this humanist genius. His brother became a surgeon, his sister married a Nobel Prize-winning physiologist. Lovingly raised, all three children never strayed far from home and the care of both parents. Keynes was damned with poor health but compensated with brilliance in mathematics, the classics and history, which saw him into Eton with a scholarship. In 1902 Keynes went to King's College, Cambridge, thanks to another scholarship, this one in mathematics, even though the true love of his life was philosophy and history. He was an active member of the Apostles (22), as well as one of the original members of the Bloomsbury Set. His family love instilled an eternal optimism in Keynes, self-confidence and the belief that man could do good and that governments could and must come to the aid of its citizens. He began publishing his first articles on economics in 1909, at age 26, and in 1911 became editor of *The Economic Journal*. He accepted a government position in the Treasury in 1915 and gave lectures. At Versailles, at the end of the First World War, he fought to prevent the allies' demands for German compensation that he knew would destroy the German people, a fight he lost, which led, first, to his resignation from the Treasury and, second, W.W. II.

In 1919 he became chairman of the British Bank of Northern Commerce in exchange for working one morning per week, at a salary of £2,000, £95,000 today]. Keynes wrote that the purpose of work was to provide leisure, and felt that everyone should work fewer hours and have longer vacations.

At the height of the Great Depression he wrote *The Means to Prosperity*, based on the need for government public spending, a copy of which went to Franklin Roosevelt, and Keynesian became the adjective applied to all new economic ideas. Without government intervention to increase expenditures, insisted Keynes, low employment would continue.

Keynes suffered a first heart attack in 1937 at age 54.

His contribution to W.W. II came in his 1940 book *How to Pay for the War* in which he recommended higher taxation, compulsory savings [the money thereby lent to the government], and the dampening of domestic demand, which would lead to less inflation, and industrial production would be diverted to the war effort and not into domestic households. After the war the money the public had stashed away in government bonds and banks would serve to insure an economic boom, which is precisely what took place. Keynes was given a seat as one of the directors of the Bank of England, as well as a hereditary peerage that came with another seat, this one in the House of Lords. At Bretton Woods Keynes argued for a world currency, the bancor, and a world central bank, ideas overruled by Americans, although the International Monetary Fund was established as a compromise.

Keynes was circumcised, the reason being the Masturbation Panic described in detail in another chapter of this book. The foreskin and its movement up and down the glans was blamed for drawing a boy's attention to his penis, leading to masturbation and the mental and physical illnesses that followed. Keynes went under the knife at age 8, an incredibly painful procedure, the agony lasting for weeks. Some doctors at the time suggested the operation be done without anesthetic, as the boy would then identify the pain as a punishment for touching the penis. When Keynes was 11 his father had the pockets of his overcoat sewn up so he couldn't fondle himself [his father confided to his diary], and most probably those of his trousers too. Richard Davenport-Hines, in his *The Seven Lives of John Maynard Keynes,* states that a politician, Lord Hailsham, still remembered the pain 70 years later, the blood ''and my sense of betrayal by the adult world''. [W.H. Auden was circumcised at age 7, after which he became erotically captivated by boys who had foreskins, as was the pornography star Al Parker (12), an obsession extensively discussed in my book *Phallus*.]

Keynes's obsession with numbers pushed him to note everything. From May 1908 to February 1909, he wrote in his diary, he had 61 sexual encounters, mainly with Duncan Grant and with both Strachey brothers, Lytton and James. From February 1909 to February 1910 he had 65 encounters; 26 from February 1910 to February 1911, and 39 from February 1911 to February 1912. His diaries were heavily encoded but the following items have been deciphered: He wrote of having sex with ''a 16-year-old under Etna'' and ''the liftboy of Vauxhall''. In 1911 he had 16 C's, 4 A's and 5 W's. Encoders guess the A's were ass-contacts, the C's cocksucking and the W's wanks [jerking off] with boys/men. The baths and saunas were the easiest places to find contacts, and Keynes knew all the parks, hotels and sites where guardsmen earned extra cash. As sodomy was punishable by imprisonment, under the same law that had seen Oscar Wilde sent away, guardsmen had to be careful. When one of Keynes's favorites was found out and was dismissed from service, he took cyanide, being, apparently, *far* from the exception. The 2008 edition of *The Atlantic* stated that the compulsion to calculate everything began in childhood, when he counted and remembered the number of steps leading up to the houses on the street where he lived, as well as detailed records of his expenses and his golf scores. In his diaries he gave the initials of the men he was bedding, GLS for Lytton Strachey, DG for Grant and nicknames, Tressider for the King's college Provost J.T. Sheppard. What went on within the Bloomsbury Set was described by Keynes's biographer Robert Skidelsky as a "sexual merry-to-round". At the time, claim his friends, he was as obsessed with whom he would share an orgasm as he was later with economic affairs or philosophy. Keynes wrote this about the Bloomsbury Set, "We repudiated general rules. We repudiated customary morals, conventions and traditional wisdom. We were, in the strict sense of the term, immoralists." For Keynes self-denial was bad, self-indulgence good [which was the undercurrent of his financial policy too]. "After all," he wrote, "in the long run we're all dead."

At Keynes's passing, in 1946, he was worth £500,000 [£20 million today], and he possessed the works of Picasso, Degas, Cézanne, Modigliani, Braque and Seurat. He died of a heart attack at age 62.

[For far more, see my book *The Bloomsbury Set*.]

Jean Genet
1910-1986

Jean Genet, from *Our Lady of the Flowers*: "But at night! Fear of the guard who may suddenly flick on the light and stick his head through the grating compels me to take sordid precautions lest the rustling of the sheets draw attention to my pleasure; but though my gesture may be less noble, by becoming secret it heightens my pleasure. I dawdle. Beneath the sheet, my right hand stops to caress the absent face, and then the whole body, of the outlaw I have chosen for that evening's delight. The left-hand closes, then arranges its fingers in the form of a hollow organ which tries to resist, then offers itself, opens up, and a vigorous body, a wardrobe, emerges from the wall, advances, and falls upon me, crushes me against my straw mattress, which has already been stained by more than a hundred prisoners, while I think of the happiness into which I sink at a time when God and

His angels exist." [Genet's full life can be found in my book *French Homosexuality*.]

Truman Capote
1924-1984

In the way he had won over Brando in Japan for his tell-all published interview that deeply humiliated the actor, Capote also succeeded in getting the facts and inner thoughts of the inhabitants of Garden City, Kansas, for his masterpiece *In Cold blood.* He had started off as a leper and finished, in his own words: "Now I'm practically the mayor." *The New Yorker* serialized the book, and like the Black and White Party that celebrated its publication, New York has known no equivalent literary sensation since.

One of the killers was Perry Smith that Carson McCullers said Truman fell in love with when he saw that Smith was as short as Truman himself, his feet hardly touching the ground when he sat. When Truman told him he was homosexual Smith said, "I guess you want to kiss me. Go ahead. The guard isn't looking." "I even masturbated him that afternoon," Capote recounted to intimate friends later, apparently proud of having masturbated the man had slaughtered two children, a boy and a girl, who had had their entire lives before them [as well as killing their parents].

Capote's form of sex was masturbation, although when his first book came out he was an effeminate beauty that even Denham Fouts, called the best-kept-boy in the world due to his good looks, was said to have paid in order for Capote to join him in Paris. Capote's looks faded rapidly, and it was mostly through masturbation that most people would have sex with him, sex he nonetheless paid for. [Gore Vidal remained handsome far longer than Capote, but when it came time for him to pay for sex, he used his buying power to make the boys do what he commanded, stating that it was basis of their jobs.]

[The lives of Capote, Denham Fouts, Isherwood, Tennessee Williams and Gore Vidal can be found in my book *American Homosexual Giants*.]

Scott O'Hara
1961 - 1998

Scott O'Hara was the author of *SeXplorers: The guide to Doing It on the Road, Do it Yourself Piston Polishing, Autopornography: A Memoir of Like in the Lust Lane* and *Rarely Pure* and *Never Simple: Selected Essays of Scott O'Hara*. His films include *Winner takes All, Below the Belt* and *In Your Wildest Dreams.* Unlike Al Parker who hated his pseudonym, Scott chose the name and loved it, and of his career he said that doing porn ''was a sheer delight from the word go''.

Like Al Parker and Casey Donovan, sex for Scott was 24/7 from the age of 15 when he wrote that he had quasi-raped a guy 28. Also like Parker, he loved saunas and backrooms, and was especially excited by public sex in parks. Again like Parker, he loved auto-fellatio. ''I got fucked almost every night, sometimes more than once. And I loved it,'' a quote brought to us by Jeffrey Escoffier.

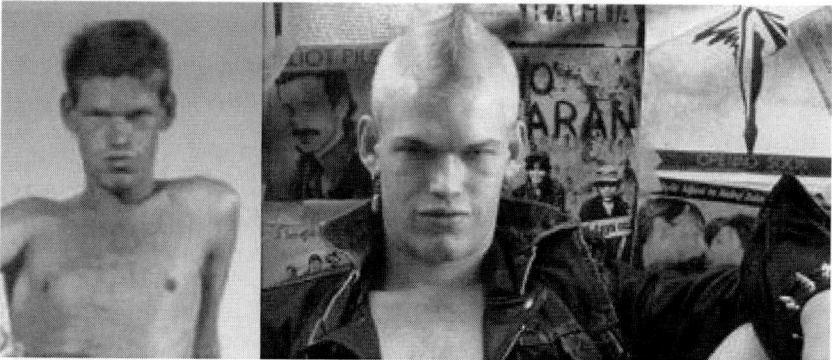

Scott O'Hara [sorry for the atrocious quality of the pics]

Scott O'Hara can write. His autobiography *Autopornography*, 1997, from which I will be quoting at length, is perfect and complete, in that Scott doesn't avoid the essential part of his life, his adolescence, the major segment of which centered around ''a horny kid, without any available outlet for your frustrated libido except your fist.'' Born in Applegate Valley in wonderfully-beautiful southern Oregon, he was a midnight jogger, whose thoughts turned to his high-school locker room where the star athlete was his idol and the Italian Aiassa brothers possessors of dicks so enormous Scott would pull over and jerk off against some tree while picturing them, so many times he'd arrive back home worn out, instantly falling into the hands of Morpheus. His mind was wild with sex, but like me in neighboring Utah, the only visible reality of his want, besides voyeurism in the daily gym class, was his collection of swimwear catalogues.

His upbringing seems to me perfect beyond words. His parents were financially independent, neither worked, his dad ''always available''. They lived on a huge farm of scenic beauty, and his brothers and he didn't sleep in beds but camped out every night in sleeping bags while Dad instructed them in constellations and the history of flying saucers. There was no television, Scott's family the only one that didn't possess one, and they basically lived on macaroni, vegetables and fruit Scott's mother jarred. He and his brothers and sisters spent enormous amounts of time in reading, and when the family was off to church on Sundays Scott cared for his aquariums and jerked off. He seems to have not been obliged to do anything he didn't wish to, like go to church.

At age 15 he seduced a man of 28 who, when he saw the 9 inches Scott was packing, begged Scott to screw him, which Scott did. He bicycled from Oregon to San Francisco to be with the guy who had taken his virginity, although the details of his deflowering are not given. He was apparently saddened by the fact that the men in San Francisco left him untouched, fearing his status as underage jailbait. He cycled to Sacramento where he allowed himself to be picked up: '' 'Do you, uh, go for guys?' I said I thought I did.'' They jerked off together, which left Scott unsatisfied, but a few minutes later he found a replacement with whom he spent the night. The next day he was picked up by some hippies, one of whom took him for a hike in the mountains to have sex: ''I just remember being incredibly happy while he was moving in me, and the birds were singing around us.''

He biked to Cheyenne where he was picked up by a boy still in high school, and then by an older man who took him home, but Scott was obliged to hide in the basement when the guy's lover unexpectedly showed up. Picked up by a guy in Nebraska, he told the man he'd never been screwed before which "turned him on like gangbusters. He was damned good at it, too--when he finished with me, I knew I'd been fucked, and I slept like a baby."

He exchanged his bike for a motorcycle, on which he discovered bathhouses, "Imagine: a milieu where sex is unabashedly the goal, the reason why everyone was there. It took my breath away."

A straight-A student, he was offered a scholarship to the University of Dallas, where sex was plentiful: "I could count on going home with someone and getting fucked. Sometimes we didn't even have to go home." One of his college tricks invited him to his apartment where he put on a porn flick. Scott had jerked off over everything from swimwear to passages from books that only had to mention a guy taking off his clothes to go for a swim in order for Scott shoot an instant load. So when the guy put on the flick, the first Scott had ever seen, he immediately jerked off, and didn't stop the rest of the night, stating that he had no idea what became of his friend. Afterwards, in bathhouses, the attraction was the videoroom where he'd do nothing but jerk off, again and again, to films he lists, my personal favorites also, like *These Basis Are Loaded* and *Inches*.

He left the university after a year and went to San Francisco where he became hooked on live jerk-off shows that he frequented as a customer until they had an amateur night. He climbed on stage and shot a load, after which the manager offered him a job that Scott immediately accepted, work he did for the next five years, four shows a week, starting at $25 and ending at $75 a show, the real money coming from what he did to the clients on a personal level, all of which led to his first film offer.

He worked up to big productions like *The Other Side of Aspen 2* where he met Al Parker, over whose filmed image he'd jerked off numerous times. Al invited him home with a friend and while Scott nailed the friend Al nailed him, a sandwich Scott appreciated. He did *Below the Belt* with David Ashfield in which both penetrated Michael Cummings at the same time. "One could always count on David for a constant hard-on," wrote Scott.

As for Scott O'Hara, he was a brilliant straight-A student, as said, a wonderful writer, a boy who, barely pubescent, made no secret of his homosexuality, which means he had great courage to face the condemnation of the religious members of the community in which he lived. He could have had all the sex his heart and body desired while succeeding in any career he may have chosen, so why he dropped his studies, studies guaranteed by a scholarship, and why he didn't turn to writing earlier, is a mystery and is our loss. Scott O'Hara died from the gay plague at age 36.

[More on Scott's life, as well as many other pornstars can be found in my book *All-Male Pornography*.]

Jack Wrangler
1946-2009

Jack Wrangler [John Robert Stillman] has a cameo role in *Kansas City Trucking Co.* In the film Boyd jerks off dreaming about Wrangler, an immensely important person in homosexual pornography. Jack Wrangler's father was the producer of such television hits as *Rawhide* and *Bonanza*. He knew he was gay at age 10, and in 1968 graduated with a degree in theater from Northwestern University, Illinois. He wanted to break into films but could only get work as a model and dancer. Born in California, he went to N.Y. where he was a bartender and go-go dancer, with the accompanying backstage hustling. He went into porn films, doing a total of 47, of which his masturbation in *Kansas City Truck Co.* was one. He wrote his autobiography and in 1976 fell in love with singer Margaret White, 22 years older than he. He cheated on her with boys and she put his bags outside their home each time, until he finally told her he'd remain faithful, after which "my sex life became very masturbatory. And I'm good at that--very good at that, in fact." [For his full life, see my book *All-Male Pornography*.]

Rich Merritt
1967 -

Few men have had sex lives as complicated as Rich Merritt's, a Marine, as disclosed in his book *Secrets of a Gay Marine Porn Star*. At age 23 Rich, still a virgin, found himself with a girl he was undressing while a buddy passed by his room to go to the toilet, from where he could watch Rich caressing the girl, the buddy stroking himself after having pissed. The guy then went into a nearby room where Rich could see him strip naked in preparation for a hot tub. The girl turned to Rich and asked him what he had in mind. ''I'm going to fuck you,'' was his nonchalant answer, something he was more than familiar with because his Marine friends talked about little else in the locker room. She refused and dressed, leaving Rich nothing better to do than strip naked and join his friend in the tub, the friend who said he was horny as hell, having just come from trying to have sex with a prostitute who had refused his credit card. The friend placed a hand on Rich's thigh, Rich a hand on the friend's dick that immediately exploded, sending clouds of semen up through the hot-tub water.

Now, what's crazy is that Rich had not only never jerked off a guy, he had also never jerked off, period. He had heard a lot about jerking off in school, but he'd always thought it meant getting hard, the pleasure of doing so being the whole of masturbation. He had had plenty of nocturnal emissions, that he would simply wipe away in the morning, hoping his mother wouldn't see stains on his sheets and briefs. He clearly remembered dreaming about naked men, how incredibly pleasant it was to do so, and even equated the intensity of his dreams with the resulting abundance of sperm he'd find in his shorts on awaking. But he'd never had an orgasm. That he hadn't a friend who had shown him how, or that he hadn't accidently rubbed himself against his bedding to orgasm, is quite simply astonishing. And that he then went on to become a pornstar is equally so.

Errol Flynn and David Niven

As stated elsewhere, Errol Flynn and David Niven shared a home with a jack-off room, which gave onto a bedroom on the ground floor through a one-way mirror in the flooring. They chose the best-looking boys and girls and gave them the use of the bedroom while they and their pals jerked off while the couples screwed below (15).

Both men shared a boat, the *Sirocco*. Girls came aboard for free, while the boys were mostly paid or offered roles in films, and if they were boys Flynn and Niven wanted back, they really did get bit-parts for services rendered. Both Flynn and Niven most probably sold themselves too for roles while living in the Garden of Allah, but direct proof is lacking. Flynn would specialize in underage girls and boys, and even as a lad in London he would masturbate before a window that gave onto a bus stop used by school girls, which once got him arrested. As he was to say later, ''I live for, with and by my balls.''

CHAPTER TWELVE

MASTURBATION TECHNIQUES
Jelqing, Tantric and Taoist eroticism, Jackinworld.com
techniques

Jelqing

Jelqing, pronounced jel-king, is practiced 30 minutes each day for months to enlarge the penile cavities, that fill with blood, making for longer and larger erections [although many doctors warn about nerve damage]. Jelqing is also called milking and is of Arab origin, from the well-named Fertile Crescent.

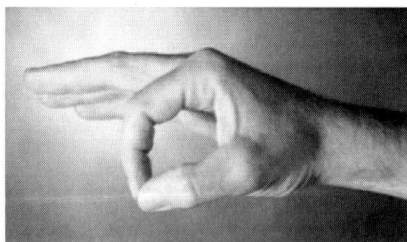

OK-grip

Form an OK-grip around the base of the phallus. With light pressure, slowly move your grip up the well-oiled shaft of the penis, stopping just before the glans. It should be done while the phallus is 50 to 100% stiff. Each repetition takes from 2-3 seconds, and after each you alternate hands. There is micro-tearing, that will increase both length and girth as it heals. For the first month use only a medium pressure grip in order to develop penis strength and resistance. Jelqing is also an exercise in self-control, not immediately cuming, restraint that will come in handy when you're in your partner.

The film by *ErosErotica,* that demonstrates jelqing, is not to be missed, and as said in the film, after the exercise the lad can reward himself with an orgasm, or save himself for his partner: https://www.pornhub.com/view_video.php?viewkey=2045336159.

Although used for penis enlargement, jelqing was nonetheless a form of masturbation, the lengthening of the member an added benefit. The risks are pain, irritation, scar formation and blood vessel tears, warn some doctors. One source I read stated that the origin goes back to when warriors had to have genitalia capable of withstanding hard pulling, without answering the question, What in the hell for?!?!

Tantric and Taoist eroticism

Tantric and Taoist eroticism means control over one's sexual energy, increasing one's erotic sensitivity without ejaculation. Self-stimulation in Tantric and Taoist eroticism is a natural part of one's being, there is nothing shameful in it, as in Western culture, where a boy is warned against masturbation, and he is not only forced to perform it hidden away in a locked bedroom or bathroom, but must do it rapidly, in order to escape detection. For Taoists, masturbation is a means of fortifying one's genitalia and amplifying one's sexual energy. Through Tantric exercises one does both, without ejaculation and loss of semen that exhaust men's vital reserves. One fully caresses one's body, nipples, scrotum, perineum, frenulum and the full length of one's penis, bringing oneself close to ejaculation several times, then stopping. You feel not only peaceful, as though you had ejaculated, but your body will be full of vigor and energy. Having an ejaculation leaves one tired and wishing to sleep, the reason an orgasm, in French, is called *la petite mort*, the little death. If you can refrain from having an orgasm you will be keen to do sports or head for the gym, and the pent-up accumulation of desire will make you more randy when ''real'' sex takes place, what in Tantric eroticism is referred to as a means of using sexual energy to amplify love.

Here is a potpourri of techniques taken from Jackinworld.com

Jackinworld bills itself: The Ultimate Male Masturbation Resource, and it is extremely complete, despite its introductory page which needs a serious face-lifting:
http://www.jackinworld.com/techniques

A few weeks ago for the first time I tried the "Backhand" grip. I had always masturbated with my right hand in the conventional way, using lube as always. When I started using my left hand, the feeling was incredible. The sensations on the head of my penis were out of this world. I could stroke up and down my penis, and at the same time, stroke in circles. This drove me insane! I had an amazing orgasm using the Backhand grip with my left hand.
Age 17

This is what I was doing in junior high: Lying on pillows and rubbing against them. I would take 2 or 3 pillows, lay them on a blanket on the floor, take off all my clothes, lie down on them, hug them, rub against them, and have amazing orgasms. I guess it was so intense because the head of my penis was being rubbed on top by the skin of my belly, and by the smooth fabric underneath. I would rub until orgasm and then lie there and hug the pillows until I was ready to go again. When I began ejaculating I had to stop doing it that way, though, because it was too much of a mess--and the older I got the less time I had to clean up. Still I do it every once in a while when I'm feeling luxurious.

The most intense, totally erotic feelings happen when I wet the end of my penis with saliva and rub the head of it--right underneath where my foreskin connects to it, near the slit. I rub it until pre-cum begins to flow--and when that happens, I spread the pre-cum all around the head but focus on the part of the head right near the slit. With my other hand I rub on the base of my penis, and I alternate rubbing the head and the base fast. When I get close to orgasm, I slow down and rub both very slowly until the pre-orgasm feeling goes away. I try to do this for at least 20 or 30 minutes. When I let myself orgasm it's pretty intense, and there is a lot more semen than if I just go for it in the usual fashion.
Age 17

I know it's kind of weird, but I am rather flexible, and I am able to perform auto-fellatio [oral stimulation of one's own penis]. It gives me all the sensations of receiving oral sex, and there's no messy cleanup. Also, it helps "train" me to prevent me from being too sensitive when I am with a girl.
Age 20

I just lube up with plenty of moisturizer and stroke my penis vigorously in front of the window. Being an exhibitionist is also a huge turn-on for me. Be more relaxed!

Age 15

I like to take a lubricated condom and put a good amount of lotion in it. Then I slip it over my penis. It slides up and down smoothly--it almost feels like a vagina. This technique creates an awesome orgasm, and it's easy to clean up. Just pull off the condom and throw it away.

Age 22

The best feeling I get is if a friend [male or female] does it for me. Another good way is lying on my back with plenty of lube. I masturbate normally; the lube just gives me a hand.

Age 15

Simply put, fast and furious. I enjoy a good, long, slow session sometimes--but going fast is the best and most intense sensation.

Age 14

I am uncircumcised, so I place my index finger and middle finger firmly on the underside of my penis [along the urethra] just under the head, with my thumb firmly on the top of my penis. I then move the foreskin back and forth over the head, using my fingers on the foreskin to massage the head. As I become aroused I start to produce "pre-cum," which mostly all stays under my skin and gets everything nice and slick. As my foreskin repeatedly covers and uncovers the head, it stimulates my frenulum and the entire head. On some strokes, but not all, I draw my snug skin completely off the head and over the corona. This has been my favorite technique since I started masturbating when I was about 10 years old. It's very simple and very intense because it has maximum stimulation of the frenulum and glans. It feels great.

Age 29

The ''Backhand''--ooh, baby!

Age 19

The Backhand is shown on a video on *Wikipedia*: Masturbation Techniques--the backhand method:

https://en.wikipedia.org/wiki/File:Masturbation_Techniques_-_the_backhand_method_(animated).gif

I *love* anal stimulation. The rubbing of my prostate enhances the whole experience tenfold--I would recommend it to anyone. This doesn't mean I am gay--only that I have found new ways to have fun with my body. It may seem weird, especially at such a young age, but I have no problem with it. Just make sure to use enough lube--it will only help your orgasm.

Age 15

I get the best sensation when I let my penis get erect for 30 to 45 minutes without touching it, just staring at it. Then I start masturbating and try to masturbate for as long as I can. I find it gives me the best orgasm.

Age 17

CHAPTER THIRTEEN

THE FIRST TIME
Mutual Masturbation and Second Orgasms

According to boys who submitted their first-time orgasms to the excellent website Jackinworld.com, a large number seemed to have had a first--and highly unexpected--orgasm alone, a self-discovery which often takes place in the shower, where soaping up their erect penises feels so good that they don't stop until they spurt their first cum. It's then that many link the event to stories they had heard, but not fully understood, related by locker-room pals.

But first we'll begin with my own first time, as related in my autobiography, *Michael Hone: His World, His Loves:* One hot August afternoon I entered his house in the middle of a football match Al was watching, his hand absently fondling himself through the extended fabric. My eye caught Nick leaning into the kitchen sink, his hand at the fly of his open levis. At first I thought he was taking a leak, but then I saw his prick out, steel hard. "What's he doing?" I murmured to Al. "Beaten' off," came the unruffled answer. "I've told you about it a dozen times, numb nuts." As I neared the kitchen, Nick turned to give me a better view, totally at ease. The top buttons of Nick's shirt were open, and while he manipulated himself with his right hand, his left was rotating over his nipples. Eventually he turned back to the basin, heaving sighs while his buttocks pushed his rod in and out of his hand, and his chest heaved out like a swimmer swimming the butterfly. Momentarily he'd pause to rub a viscous substance, secreted by the piss hole, over the head. The operation brought on even deeper moans. At times he'd stop, as if to catch his breath, then he'd start up again, then stop, then begin again until he suddenly fell forward like a puppet cut from its strings, while jet after jet of a white substance pulsed into the basin and onto the wall beyond. I stepped back in surprise, while Al whooped from his place on the sofa. Although I was rock-hard myself, there was no question of exposing my boyhood to be compared to Nick's incredible tool. So I ran home to try out the experience on myself, to its blissful and natural end for the first time.

I imagine that a boy's first time often takes place like this: Let me say first that I do not masturbate, the term masturbation indicates something that society has made ugly. Personally, I jack off. [Something to which the author fully subscribes.] The first time I jacked off was with my best friend Allen. He and I were 12 or 13 at that time. Allen had gone to his cousin's house for the weekend, and the next time we got together he showed me what he had learned from his cousin. Well, that was the first time I jacked off and I have enjoyed it ever since. From that time until I went away to college, Allen and I spent a number of weekends a month together, either at his house or mine, and we jacked off together every time. I never thought anything about us jacking off together; it just seemed perfectly natural. We were best friends and we were sharing a good time."

A boy of 11 records meeting up with a friend who had gotten hold of a porno film and, along with a buddy, they went to the guy's home to watch it. ''We were all hornier than ever, and somebody suggested that we whip them out and go for it. We all did, and even though I had never jacked off before, I knew what to do from watching them. I never had an orgasm, but later that week I tried it again in my bedroom.'' He got naked and massaged his cock and balls. ''I remember moving my foreskin back and forth over the head slowly for 5 or 10 minutes. I started speeding up and was suddenly filled with an amazing pleasurable sensation. Nothing came out, but I knew it was my first orgasm.''

Another boy noticed how big a guy's dick was in his high school showers. The guy was uncut, and one day walking home together the boy asked to see it. This led to a jerking-off session, which led to mutual masturbation and ''docking'' [the boy's cut glans introduced into the guy's foreskin]. ''He introduced me to jerking off with lube, because that's how he did it. He laid me down on the floor once and used oil as he stroked me. It gave me one of the best orgasms of my life. Of course, I returned the favor.''

During a sleepover a friend asked me, ''Do you know what masturbation is?'' ''Isn't that what happens when a woman has her period?'' ''No, stupid, that's menstruation. I'm talking about something that makes you feel good.'' We went into the bathroom and Tim removed his briefs and stood in front of the sink. He took some soap and lathered his hands. He put the soap onto his penis and started to jerk off. I stood there not knowing what to do, but finally I joined in. Tim kneeled on the floor and continued to jerk off. I kneeled alongside him and after a few minutes he began to groan. Then he shot some white stuff onto the floor. I continued to masturbate. After what couldn't have been more than 30 seconds, my body shuddered. My first orgasm.

A boy in the 7th grade went to a friend's birthday party during which a porno film was put on, the first the boy had seen. He watched his friends fiddling with their dicks inside their jeans and when he asked what they were doing, one said, beating the meat. He went home and tried it, but nothing happened other than it felt good. Two weeks later his friend invited him back to his house where he put on a hard-core film. The boy saw that just fiddling with a penis wasn't enough, it had to be stroked. Back home he tried it that way, and had his first orgasm. ''What came out of my penis was a sticky whitish liquid. I wiped it up and decided that this was the greatest thing that had ever happened to me.''

When I was 10, I was spending the night at my friend Kent's house. We were in a ''tent'' in his living room that he'd made out of blankets. While there, he asked, ''Wanna know something that feels really good?'' Of course I said, ''Yes''.
Kent pulled down his shorts and underwear, placing his fingers over and around his penis. Neither of us had started puberty. He said, 'You pull up and down on your wiener like this'.
I pulled down my clothes too, and began to mimic his actions. I didn't really get it at first, but after a while it gave me a warm, tingly feeling that I liked.
Following that, we sometimes did it together, and I occasionally did it on my own. It wasn't that often, until my testicles grew and began producing testosterone. Then I felt a stronger desire to do it.

It was some time before I had my first weak orgasm. I still didn't associate the act with anything "sexual". It wasn't until I began to ejaculate, at age 12, that I figured out my actions in some way related to what I'd learned about reproduction.

Then I felt guilty for what had just felt good before. I wish my dad or older brother had talked to me about sex in general and masturbation in particular. It would have prevented a lot of guilt feelings and weird ideas I had.

Mutual Masturbation

Two additional texts about mutual jerking off: My girlfriend is used to it now, she knows I wank a lot and she came home from work a couple of times and caught me and my mate James in the middle of it, watching porn and wanking off on the couch. She freaks out about it and complains about finding tissues and stuff but when we're horny she says she gets turned on thinking about me watching my mates cum. She wants to have a threeway at some time but I ain't sure about that.

I've only wanked other lads off a few times. But I still don't think that's a big deal either, we've both got cocks and we're both having a wank so what difference does it make if we wank each other? I know I'm not interested in sucking dick or butt fucking or anything like that, it's just a couple of mates working on their cocks and having a laugh.

Second Orgasms

I masturbate in about 10 minutes--that's from being naked with an erection to orgasm. I usually stroke it as fast as I can because it feels so good. Sometimes it takes longer but sometimes I shoot in just a minute or two. I don't want to climax faster, but I wish the orgasm would last longer! Or it would be nice if I could do it again right away. A few times my penis stayed erect so I kept stroking, and in 10-15 minutes had a really intense second orgasm. [Age 15]

CHAPTER FOURTEEN

MASTURBATION IN LITERATURE, SONGS AND VIDEOS

Literature

The book *Alcibiades the Schoolboy* was originally written in Italian by Antonio Rocco, in 1630, and then translated into French by, *perhaps*, Édouard Cléder. Due to the expense of the English version--when found--I decided to translate it myself from the French, my second language, into English, my first. I've at times inserted the French translation so that Francophiles can follow the text in the original.

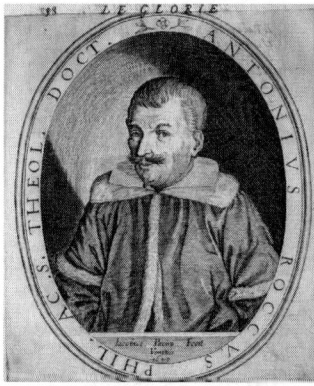

Antonio Rocco

Incredibly, Rocco was a priest, as well as a writer and Aristotelian philosophy teacher. He wrote *Alcibiades the School Boy* in 1630. It's first publication, in 1652, was destroyed due to the filth of its content, all but a few surviving copies, and was republished in 1862. It was again found filthy and again largely destroyed. It is one of the earliest texts on masturbation, Rocco's argument taken up by Tissot two hundred years later. Philotime is modeled after Socrates and the text is considered the world's first homoerotic novel.

''Before going further with me, my master, please satisfy my curiosity on other points. If one doesn't wish to go with women or boys, can one not assuage his ardors by himself with his own hands, without spending money, without fatigue, without submitting to anyone? Thanks to this means, we have immediate and infallible remedy for each and every sensual itch.''

''Alcibiades my belovèd, jerking yourself with your own hands (*se pomper les humeurs avec ses propres mains*) is a miserable expedient which deprives us of our true being and kills our passion for the real thing. It's not only our semen that comes out, it's our very blood. It alters our features, makes us pale, and can even hasten death. Nature puts everything in the preparation of our dew, for it is that which regenerates our species. She makes it with the purest part of our blood, an enterprise that weakens our veins and saps the vital parts of our bodies. If we satisfy ourselves with our hands it becomes a habit thanks to the ease of doing so. Whereas pleasure we have with the person we love calms our spirit and contents our desire. Jerking leaves us unfulfilled and tires us out because, due to its facility, we do it so often.''

[The full life of Alcibiades, as well as the translation of Rocco's book into English, can be found on Amazon: Michael Hone/*Alcibiades the School Boy*.]

Whereas Jean-Jacque Rousseau found autoerotism ''a dangerous supplement,'' the philosopher Denis Diderot wrote, in 1782, ''It is a need and a sweet thing. It is a call from Nature to help it, and although we will not provoke it, let us lend it a helping hand, occasionally. I see only foolish, wasted pleasure in denying it.'' Diderot went on to confess: ''My father's page boys taught me through kindness.'' For the Marquis de Sade, imprisoned for 30 years, autoerotism was the supreme pleasure: ''He was jerking off. I watched the voluptuous sensation carrying him entirely out of himself, his moans, his groans, his strokes as he reached the very last stages of pleasure, and I saw his tool spill sperm in the same vase I'd just filled.''

Psychiatrist and sexologist Philippe Brenot, author of *In Praise of Masturbation*, brings us this quote from Apollinaire, *The Debauched Hospodar*, 1907, ''He started to masturbate them [2 girls], each with one hand, while they were exciting his cock.'' And on the Orient Express Apollinaire was relieved by his manservant: ''Cornaboeux's fingers delicately unbuttoned the prince's trousers. They took hold of the delirious penis which on all accounts justified the famous couplet by Alphonse Allais: 'The exciting vibration of trains/Slides desire into the marrow of our loins.' ''

Writer Michel Tournier wrote *The Meteors*: ''The brain provides the sexual organ with an imaginary object. This object rests with the hand to embody it. The hand is the ideal partner. Like an actor the hand plays the role it is given, but its masterpiece is masturbation. There it becomes at will either a penis or a vagina.'' Guillaume Fabert wrote in *Self-portrait of an Erection*, masturbation ''is to sex what aspirin is to medicine: *panacea*.''

Chuck Palahniuk wrote *Fight Club* from which the Norton/Pitt film was made. He also did a video/soliloquy on masturbation called *Guts*, twenty-one very strange minutes, seen on YouTube. https://www.youtube.com/watch?v=EL20eY34kmE

Bernard Lefkowitz wrote *Our Guys*, about high school athletes who gang-raped a girl with a minimal IQ. What is striking about the boys is their incredible beauty and the variety of their sex, going from intercourse and blow jobs to hiding out in a friend's closet while he screwed a girl, jumping out in the middle, the guy doing the screwing not even caring if the girl left in a huff. The boys were so cute--one of whom, the star athlete, was promised to girls in order to get them to one of his friend's homes, who filled in when the cutie didn't show up--that they didn't have to rely on girls with low IQs, but so bored that they graduated to the use of baseball bats and broomsticks to prod vaginas. "On nonpractice afternoons, some of the Jocks would gather at a house where the parents were gone and watch porn, as they all masturbated together" and it was rumored that they "stood in a circle watching a porn movie, each jerking off onto a slice of bread." "The Jocks found pornography exciting because it could be shared by the entire viewing audience. It wasn't an individual experience. It was group onanism." "The devotion to activities such as circle-jerks, 'voyeuring', oral sex performed by one girl on a number of guys, watching pornography together may suggest a homoerotic tendency among members of the adolescent male groups that become involved in sexual assaults. In the Glen Ridge group, homoeroticism may have been a factor," but it was also a way of "impressing your friend with your sexual prowess. A group of appreciative and responsive buddies is essential to build a reputation for sexual control and domination."

Songs

Best song on masturbation: *Get a Grip* [on Yourself] by Semisonic on YouTube.

https://www.youtube.com/watch?v=jrdZNNG4S8g

John Strachan is a song writer. His father made his fortune in trading horses, a trade Strachan, 1875-1958, continued. He organized dances at his farms in Scotland, some that attracted the attention of American producers who invited him to the States to perform, although he refused. Some of his songs are bawdy, like The *Ball of Kirriemuir*:

The elders of the church
They were too old to firk [fuck]
So they sat around the table
And had a circle jerk.

A hardcore punk band called the Bedwetters came out with a first album they called Group Sex. In 1979 the name of the group was changed to Circle Jerks by vocalist Keith Morris.

Videos

1- Blake Mitchell of Helix does a 1-minute how-best-to-jack-off video, found on Pornhub: Blake Mitchell Experiencing a Complete [uncut dick] Orgasm.
   https://www.pornhub.com/view_video.php?viewkey=ph5aa5 464435f5e

2- XTAPES.TO brings us a great video showing Cody Cummings jerking off Donny Wright. Called: Master Masseur--Cody Cummings & Donny Wright.
   http://gay.xtapes.to/master-masseur-cody-cummings-donny-wright-2012/

3- In a locker room 2 guys masturbate in front of each other. First rate.
   https://fr.xhamster.com/videos/a-pair-of-wankers-5011782#mlrelated

4- Christian St John locker-room solo
   https://www.xnxx.com/video-2dub164/christian_st_john

5- A wonderful mutual jerk off in *El Paso Wrecking Corp*, found, among other sites, on Redtube, at minute 15 of the 46-minute scene: https://fr.redtube.com/184804.

6- *Kansas City Trucking Co.* is all about masturbation, which director Joe Gage explains in this way: ''The whole idea of making homosexual pornography [if] you strip it down to its absolute basics, is the worship of the phallus, the worship of the penis (4). If you're going to make homosexual pornography, you'd better light the dick. You're highlighting the penis--that's what it's about.'' Found on Boyfriendtv: https://www.boyfriendtv.com/videos/86054/kansas-city-trucking-co/?m=1

7- J. Brian, producer and director, is a man we know literally nothing about, but he was the creator of *Seven in a Barn*, a homoerotic classic: One of the opening scenes in *Seven in a Barn* has the boys in the midst of a poker game, the winner becoming the master of the other six boys present, the loser the boys' slave. The loser happens to be both the oldest boy and the best looking, the master a beautiful ''all boy'' swimmer-body type, who orders the slave to do what the boys want, beginning with commands given by the first boy, chosen because he has the biggest dick, then the second boy, chosen because he has the biggest balls, the third boy, who has the second-biggest dick, and so on. The only interdiction is that the slave can't cum, his orgasm reserved for the master himself who will have twenty minutes with him after the slave has made the other five ejaculate, some by blowing, some by fucking, some by jerking them off. The slave does cum, however, over his chest in veritable lakes, along with the two boys who had brought him off with tongues, mouths and hands.

　　The film has its place here because 90% of what goes on is masturbation in one form or another.

A Panel on Pornography was set up by the New University, Orange County California, in 1972, one of the subjects for discussion being *Seven in a Barn* and the works of J. Brian. The copy of the film was seized by Orange Country sheriffs, at first causing the students handling the film to flee, then inciting full-scale student protests. In the spring of 1971 homosexual films had already been shown at a California university in a course entitled ''Varieties of Human Sexuality,'' consisting of *L.A. Man* and *Bike Boy*. Chancellor Aldrich declared that he hadn't forbidden the screening of *Seven in a Barn*, but that the sheriff's office was ''free to act as it saw fit''. The Vice Chancellor stated that there was no place for hardcore pornography on the campus, something ''devoid of educational and artistic value''. The campus Gay Student Union answered that it was saddened that *Seven in a Barn* was labeled hardcore pornography [the reader can decide for himself]. That said, the film's a wonderful source of erotic pleasure and self-pleasuring, an *absolute must-see* for those who don't mind homoerotic goings-on (12).

https://fr.xhamster.com/videos/vintage-j-brian-1971-6436106

also:

https://sextubespot.com/videos/3176616/vintage-j-brian-1971/

8- There's a 7-minute 1997 video by Vincent Ravalec called *Portrait des hommes qui se branlent* [*The Masturbators*], which portraits the Parisian Bois de Boulogne through which women drive in usually very expensive cars, naked under their furs, who eventually pull over and allow boys to watch them stroke their naked pussies, the boys mad with lust, many cuming while running up to the cars, not even hard, the rubbing of the jeans denim enough to bring them off, while those who reach the car windows ejaculate over the glass, their cocks, all uncut, shown hard and spurting, while a film narrative accentuates what's going on, ''When you look at sperm each guy's is different, the first was completely clear, like water, and the other looked like cream, maybe having something to do with the personality of the guys or how often they yank it, in a little while the liquid gets more fluid, almost pure. When I jerk off I do it so often that I end up with aching balls. The cars that stop and the guys jerking off, out of their minds, forest Pans on the loose: O show me your breasts and your pussy too, pull down your pantyhose, watch me while I get hard.'' The film is also in book form, found on Amazon, but I'm unable to find the video on sale anywhere.

9- A San Diego Chargers Security guard caught on video masturbating a few feet away from cheerleaders jumping up and down. Unique.
https://heavy.com/sports/2016/12/san-diego-chargers-qualcomm-security-guard-masturbates-masturbating-cheerleaders-video-fired/

Three jokes to end the chapter

Dad: Hey son, if you keep masturbating you're going to go blind.
Son: Dad, I'm over here.

What do a penis and a Rubik's Cubes have in common?
The more you play with it, the harder it gets.

A 12-year-old boy heard his mom moaning and went to see why. She was in bed naked, rubbing herself and saying, ''I need a man, I need a man.'' A week later he heard her moaning again, but in a different way. He looked in her room and saw her with a man. He ran back into his room, stripped naked and rubbed himself where she'd been rubbing, while pleading, ''I need a bike, I need a bike.''

CLOSING DEDICATION

I wish to end this book with a dedication to Matthew Burdette--a high school Boy Scout, wrestler and member of the polo team--who was surreptitiously filmed while masturbating in the school john, by a fellow student who posted it on the Net. Ruthlessly teased, he wrote in his suicide note, ''I have no friends. I don't want to kill myself but I have no friends.'' He was 14.

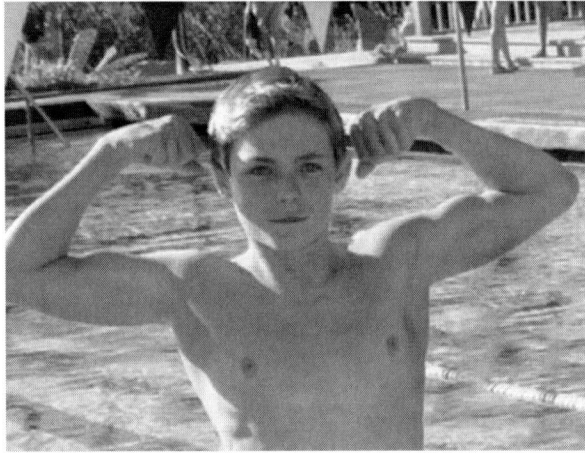

SOURCES

(1) See my book *Omnisexuality, The Death of Gay and Straight Sex*.
(2) See my book *SPARTA*.
(3) See my book *Omnisexuality* for details.
(4) See my book *Phallus*.
(5) See my book *Roman Homosexuality*.
(6) See my book *Greek Homosexuality*.
(7) See my book *The History of British Homosexuality*.
(8) See my book HUSTLERS.
(9) See my book *The History of Orgies*.
(10) See my book *American Homosexual Giants*.
(11) See my book *The Bloomsbury Set*.
(12) See my book *All-Male Pornography*.
(13) See my book *German Homosexuality*.
(14) See my autobiography, *Michael Hone, His World, His Loves*.
(15) See my book *Garden of Allah*.
(16) See my book *Boarding School Homosexuality*.

(17) See my book *RENT BOYS*.
(18) See my book *The Belle Epoque*.
(19) See my book *The Essence of Being Gay*.
(20) See my book *Capri Homosexual Paradise*.
(21) See my book *French Homosexuality*.
(21) See my book *John (Jack) Nicholson*.
(22) See my book *Homosexual Secret Societies*.

Aggleton, Peter, *Men Who Sell Sex*, 1999.
Aldrich and Wotherspoon, *Who's Who in Gay and Lesbian History*, 2001.
Aldrich, Robert, *The Seduction of the Mediterranean*, 1993.
Alexander The Great, edited by Heckel and Tritle, 2009.
Baker Simon, *Ancient Rome*, 2006.
Beachy, Robert, *Gay Berlin*, 2014. Marvelous.
Boswell, John, *Christianity, Social Tolerance, and Homosexuality*, 1980.
Boswell, John, *Same-Sex Unions*, 1994.
Bowers, Scotty, *Full Service*, 2012.
Bret, David, *Errol Flynn, Gentleman Hellraiser*, 2004,
Bret, Davis, *Trailblazers*, 2009.
Bull, Lew, *Memoirs of a Hustler*, 2010.
Burg, B.R., *Gay Warriors*, 2002.
Burg, B.R., *Sodomy and the Pirate Tradition*, 1989.
Bury and Meiggs, *A History of Greece*, 1975.
Calimach, Andrew, *Lover's Legends*, 2002.
Carpenter, Edward, *The Intermediate Sex*, 1912.
Carson, H.A., *a thousand and one night stands*, 2001.
Carter, William, *Proust in Love*, 2006.
Cavel Benjamin, *Rumble, Young Man, Rumble*, 2003.
Cawthorne, Nigel, *Sex Lives of the Popes*, 1996
Clark, Adrian and Jeremy Dronfield, *Queer Saint, Peter Watson*, 2015.
Clark, Gerald, *Capote*, 1988.
Crompton, Louis, *Homosexuality and Civilization*, 2003.
Crowley, Roger, *Empires of the Sea*, 2008. Marvelous.
Davenport-Hines, Richard, *The Seven Lives of Maynard Keynes*, 2015.
Davidson, James, *Courtesans and Fishcakes*, 1998.
Davidson, James, *The Greeks and Greek Love*, 2007.
Davidson, Michael, *The World, The Flesh and Myself*, 1977.
Dorais, Michel, *Rent Boys*, 2002.
Dover K.J. *Greek Homosexuality*, 1978
Edmonson, Roger, *CLONE, The Life and Legend of Al Parker*, 2000.
Eisler, Benita, *BYRON Child of Passion, Fool of Fame*, 2000. Wonderful.
Ellmann, Richard, *Oscar Wilde*, 1987.
Erlanger, Philippe, *The King's Minion*, 1901.

Escoffier, Jeffrey, *Bigger Than Life*, 2009.
Everitt, Anthony, *Hadrian*, 2009.
Fagles, Robert, *The Iliad*, 1990.
Fox, Robin Lane, *Alexander the Great*, 1973.
Fraser, Antonia, *The Gunpowder Plot*, 1996.
Gathorne-Hardy, Jonathan, *The Public School Phenomenon*, 1977.
Gidel, Henry, *Cocteau*, 2009.
Gillman, Peter and Leni, *The Wildest Dream*, 2000.
Gilmore, John, *Laid Bare*, 1997.
Gilmore, John, *Live Fast—Die Young*, 1997.
Graham, Robb, *Strangers*, 2003.
Grant Michael, *History of Rome*, 1978
Graves, Robert, *Greek Myths*, 1955.
Guicciardini, *Storie fiorentine (History of Florence)*, 1509. Essential.
Halperin David M. *One Hundred Years of Homosexuality*, 1990
Harris, Frank, *My Life and Loves*, 1925.
Hibbard, Allen, *Paul Bowles*, 1993.
Hibbert, Christopher, *Florence, the Biography of a City*, 1993.
Hickman, Tom, *God's Doodle--The Life and Times of the Penis*, 2012.
Hirst, Michael, *The Tudors*, 2007.
Hofler, Robert, *Party Animals,* 2010.
Hogan, Steve, *Completely Queer, Gay and Lesbian Encyclopedi*a, 1998.
Holroyd, Michael, *Lytton Strachey*, 1994.
Hughes Robert, *Rome*, 2011
Hughes-Hallett, *Heroes*, 2004.
Isherwood, Charles, *The Life and Death of Joey Stefano*, 1996.
Isherwood, Christopher, *Christopher and His Kind*, 1976.
Isherwood, Christopher, *Diaries*, vol. one, 2011.
James, Callum, *My Dear KJ...* edited by James, 2015.
Jouhandeau, Marcel, *Ecrits secrets*, 1988.
Katz, Jonathan Ned, *Love Stories*, 2001.
Kearns, Michael, *The Truth is Bad Enough*, 2012,
Kelly, Ian, *Casanova: Actor Lover Priest Spy*, 2008.
Knights, Sarah, *Bloomsbury's Outside, A Life of David Garnett*, 2015.
Korda, Michael, *HERO The Life and Legend of Lawrence of Arabia*, 2010.
Lahr, John, *Prick Up Your Ears, The Biography of Joe Orton*, 1978
Lahr, John, *Tennessee Williams, Mad Pilgrimage of the Flesh*, 2014.
LaRue, Chi Chi, *Making it Big*, 1997.
Lefkowitz, Bernard, *Our Guys*, 1997.
Livy, *Rome and the Mediterranean*
Lubkin, Gregory, *A Renaissance Court*, 1994.
Lyons, Mathew, *The Favourite*, 2011.
Mackay, John Henry, *The Hustler*, 2002.

Manchester, William, *A World Lit Only By Fire*, 1993.
Mann, William, *Men Who Love Men*, 2007.
Mann, William, *The Men from the Boys*, 1998.
Mann, William, *Wisecracker*, 1998.
Manso, Peter, *Brando*, 1994.
Marchand, Leslie, *Byron*, 1971.
Maugham, Robin, *Escape from the Shadows*, 1972.
McBrien, William, *Cole Porter*, 2000.
McCann, Graham, *Rebel Males*, 1991.
McGilligan, Patrick, *A Double Life--George Cukor*, 1991.
Mercer, John, *Gay Pornography*, 2017.
Merrick/Sibalis, *Homosexuality in French History and Culture*, 2012.
Merritt, Rich, *Secrets of a Gay Marine Porn Star*, 2005.
Miles Richard, *Ancient Worlds*, 2010.
Miles Richard, *Carthage Must be Destroyed*, 2010
Minichiello, Victor and John Scott, *Male Sex Work and Society*, 2014.
Mitford, Nancy, *Frederick the Great*, 1970.
Moore Lucy, *Amphibious Thing*, 2000.
Nicholl, Charles, *The Reckoning*, 2002.
Niven, David, *Bring on the Empty Horses*, 1975.
Niven, David, *The Moon's a Balloon*, 1971.
Noel, Gerard, *The Renaissance Popes*, 2006.
Norton, Rictor, *My Dear Boy, Gay Love Letters*, 1998.
O'Donnell, *Love, Sex, Intimacy and Friendship between Men*, 2003.
O'Hara, Scott, *Autopornography, A Memoir of Life in the Lust Lane*, 1997.
O'Hara, Scott, *Do-It-Yourself Piston Polishing,* 1996.
Brenot, Philippe, *In Praise of Masturbation*, 1997.
Oosterhuis and Kennedy, *Homosexuality and Male Bonding*, 1991.
Opper Thorsten, *Hadrian*, 2008.
Ostrow, Steve, *Live at the Continental*, 2007.
Paladilhe, Dominique, *Le Prince de Condé*, 2005.
Paring, Justin, *The life and times of Samuel Steward*, 2010.
Parini, Jay, *Empire of Self, A Life of Gore Vidal*, 2015.
Parish, James Robert, *The Hollywood Book of Death,* 2002.
Parker, Peter, *Isherwood A Life*, 2004.
Pascal, Jean Claude, *L'Amant du Roi*, 1991.
Pearce, Joseph, *The Unmasking of Oscar Wilde*, 2000.
Pernot, Michel, *Henri III*, Le Roi Décrié, 2013, Excellent book.
Petitfils, Jean-Christian, *Louis XIII*, 2008.
Peyrefitte, Roger, *Propos secrets,* Volumes 1 and 2, 1977, 1980.
Plimpton, George, *Truman Capote*, 1998.
Plutarch's Lives, Modern Library.
Polybius, *The Histories*

Porter, Darwin & Roy Moseley, *Damn You, Scarlett O'Hara*, 2011.
Porter, Darwin and Danforth Prince, *Pink Triangle*, 2014.
Porter, Darwin, *Brando Unzipped*, 2004.
Porter, Darwin, *Howard Hughes*, 2010.
Rader, Dotson, *Blood Dues*, 1974.
Read, Piers Paul, *The Templars*, 1999.
Reed, Jeremy, *The Dilly*, 2014.
Reid, B.L., *The Lives of Roger Casement*, 1976.
Revenin, Régis, *Homosexualité et Prostitution Maculines à Paris*, 2005.
Robb, Graham, *Rimbaud*, 2000. Superb.
Rocco, Antonio, *Alcibiade Enfant à l'Ecole*, 1630.
Rocke, Michael, *Forbidden Friendships*, 1996. Fabulous.
Roen, Paul, *High Camp*, 1994.
Rolfe, Frederick, Letters to Charles Kains Jackson, *My Dear KJ...*, 2015.
Romans Grecs et Latin, Gallimard, 1958.
Rouse, W.H.D., Homer's *The Iliad*, 1938.
Royle, Trevor, *Fighting Mac, The Downfall of Sir Hector Macdonald*.
Ruggiero, Guido, *The Boundaries of Eros*, 1985.
Saslow, James, *Ganymede in the Renaissance*, 1986.
Saul, Jack, *The Sins of the Cities of the Plain*.
Sawyer-Lauçanno, *An Invisible Specter, Paul Bowles*, 1989.
Schama, Simon, *Citizens* 1989.
Setz, Wolfram, *The Sins of the Cities of the Plain*, 1881.
Seymour, Craig, *All I could Bare*, 2008.
Shakespeare, Nicholas, *Bruce Chatwin*, 1999.
Sharaf, Myron, *Fury on Earth: A Biography of Wilhelm Reich*, 1983.
Shaw, Aiden, *Sordid Truths*, 2009.
Shelden, Michael, *Graham Greene, The Man Within*, 1994.
Sheridan, Alan, *André Gide*, 1999.
Shilts, Randy, *And the Band Played on*, 1987.
Sipriot, Pierre, *Montherlant sans masque*, 1982.
Skidelsky, Robert, *The Essential Keynes*, 2016.
Skidmore, Chris, *Death and the Virgin*, 2010.
Soares, André, *The Life of Ramon Novarro*, 2010.
Spalding, Frances, *Duncan Grant*, 1997.
Spoto, Donald, *The Kindness of Strangers*, 1997.
Strathern, Paul, *The Medici, Godfathers of the Renaissance*, 2003. Superb.
Strauss Barry, *The Spartacus War*, 2009.
Tamagne, Florence, *A History of Homosexuality in Europe*, 2004.
Teeman, Tim, *In Bed with Gore Vidal*, 2013.
Terry, Paul, *In Search of Captain Moonlite*, 2013.
That Man: Peter Berlin, DVD.
Turnbaugh, Douglas Blair, *Duncan Grant*, 1987.

Vanderbilt, Arthur, *Best-Kept Boy in the World*, 2014.
Vernant, Jean-Pierre, *Mortals and Immortals*, 1991.
Vidal, Gore, *Palimpsest: A Memoir*, 1995.
Violet, Bernard, *Les Mystères Delon*, 2000.
Walsh, Kenneth M., *wasn't tomorrow wonderful?* 2014.
Watson, Steven, *Factory Made*, 2003.
Weinberg, Williams and Pryor, *Dual Attraction*, 1994.
Wikipedia: Research today is impossible without the aid of this monument.
Williams Craig A. *Roman Homosexuality*, 2010
Winecoff, Charles, *Anthony Perkins, split image*, 1996.
Wolff, Geoffrey, *Black Sun: The Violent Eclipse of Harry Crosby*, 1976.
Woods, Gregory, *Homintern*, 2016.
Wright, Ed, *History's Greatest Scandals*, 2006.
Zachks, Richard, *History Laid Bare*, 1994.
Zeeland, Steven, *Barrack Buddies and Soldier Lovers*, 1993.
Zeeland, Steven, *Military Trade*, 1999.
Zeeland, Steven, *Sailors and Sexual Identity*, 1995.
Zeeland, Steven, *The Masculine Marine*, 1996.

INDEX

Please note that the page numbers are *passim*. An example, fleshlight 76 – 102, means that fleshlight is found within these pages, but not necessarily on *every* page.

Made in United States
North Haven, CT
04 October 2022